THE NEW ART AND SCIENCE OF PREGNANCY AND CHILDBIRTH

What You Want
to Know from
Your Obstetrician

THE NEW ART AND SCIENCE OF PREGNANCY AND CHILDBIRTH

What You Want to Know from Your Obstetrician

Tan Thiam Chye
Tan Kim Teng
Tan Heng Hao
John Tee Chee Seng

KK Women's and Children's Hospital,
Singapore

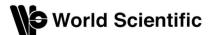

World Scientific

NEW JERSEY · LONDON · SINGAPORE · BEIJING · SHANGHAI · HONG KONG · TAIPEI · CHENNAI

Published by

World Scientific Publishing Co. Pte. Ltd.

5 Toh Tuck Link, Singapore 596224

USA office: 27 Warren Street, Suite 401–402, Hackensack, NJ 07601

UK office: 57 Shelton Street, Covent Garden, London WC2H 9HE

Library of Congress Cataloging-in-Publication Data
The new art and science of pregnancy and childbirth: what you want to know from your obstetrician/
edited by Tan Thiam Chye ... [et al.].
    p. cm.
    Includes index.
    ISBN-13: 978-981-277-939-7 (hardcover : alk. paper)
    ISBN-10: 981-277-939-6 (hardcover : alk. paper)
    ISBN-13: 978-981-277-940-3 (pbk. : alk. paper)
    ISBN-10: 981-277-940-X (pbk. : alk. paper)
    1. Pregnancy--Popular works. 2. Childbirth--Popular works. I. Tan, Thiam Chye
RG525.N386 2008
618.2--dc22

                                2007051863

British Library Cataloguing-in-Publication Data
A catalogue record for this book is available from the British Library.

Disclaimer:
This book is meant as an informational guide for readers. While all efforts have been made to verify the accuracy and consistency of the information presented, you are urged to seek professional advice for specific health needs.

Printed by Fulsland Offset Printing (S) Pte Ltd, Singapore

Foreword

66 **The New Art and Science of Pregnancy and Childbirth"** is clearly a product of the absolute dedication of a group of medical specialists, to obstetric care at the KK Women's & Children's Hospital. The myriad of writers included obstetricians, neonatologist, anesthetist, psychiatrist, sports physician, nurses, allied healthcare providers, dentist, dermatologist and a TCM physician.

This book comprehensively covered the entire spectrum of topics relating to pregnancy, starting from pre-pregnancy issues to post-delivery care.

I congratulate the editors and authors for organizing the topics systematically and in a manner as understandable by a layperson. The FAQ style makes easy reading and helps in the quick assimilation of the medical information. It informs a reader what medical caregivers look for, the rationale of care and how she can adequately prepare herself for a consultation, for her delivery or for a procedure.

This book is certainly the most updated and comprehensive book on pregnancy care written by Singapore medical specialists and caregivers. I envisage it will become an important reference book for anyone who is preparing for pregnancy or for those who are going through pregnancy.

I salute the editors and authors for their devotion to their obstetric calling at the KK Women's & Children's Hospital and the timely production of this important reading material for the public.

TAY, Eng-Hseon
Clinical Associate Professor,
Senior Consultant Gynecologist,
Chairman, Medical Board
KK Women's & Children's Hospital

Of all the rights and privileges of a woman,
The greatest is motherhood.

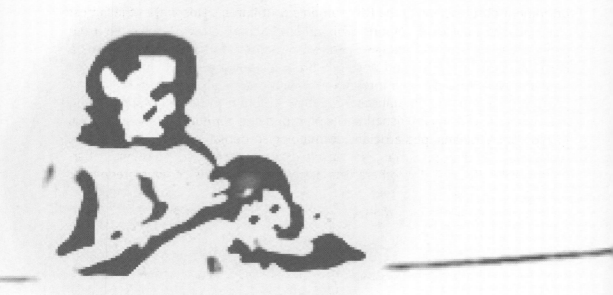

Preface

Pregnancy is a very exciting time for every woman. Feeling your baby grow inside you is a unique and wondrous experience. Many couples, however, experience some degree of anxiety and uncertainty. For some, this may be their first pregnancy. Some might have developed complications during the previous pregnancy and are worried about the current pregnancy.

Every woman wants a smooth pregnancy, easy delivery and a healthy baby. Knowing more about pre-pregnancy preparation, understanding pregnancy, birth and the small risk of complications can help to dispel worry and uncertainty. You will then be more able to make informed choices in your pregnancy. On the other hand, many mothers-to-be read about pregnancy and labor from the internet and are confused by the myriad of information that is available.

The New Art and Science of Pregnancy and Childbirth is written by prominent obstetricians in the KK Women's & Children's Hospital — the largest maternity hospital in Singapore, which delivers about 12 000 deliveries each year. It is a new art and science because the practices today are based on the latest scientific evidence and not on old wives' tales any more.

This book provides comprehensive information on pre-pregnancy care, pregnancy, delivery, postnatal care as well as confinement practices and care of the newborn. Our distinguished panel of experts who contributed to this book include obstetricians, pediatrician, dermatologist, dental surgeon, psychiatrist, traditional Chinese physician, sports physician, anesthetist, dietitians, pharmacist, midwife and physiotherapists. It covers all aspects of your pregnancy, especially in our Asian context.

Happy reading and we wish you a healthy pregnancy and baby!

Thiam Chye, TAN
MBBS (Singapore), MMed (O&G) (Singapore)

Heng Hao, TAN
MBBS (Singapore), MMed (O&G) (Singapore), MRCOG (London)

Kim Teng, TAN
MBBS (Singapore), MMed (O&G) (Singapore), MRACOG (RANZCOG), FAMS (Singapore)

John Chee Seng, TEE
MBBS (Singapore), MMed (O&G) (Singapore), FAMS (Singapore)

To friendship and our loved ones,
who add meaning to our lives.

To all our patients,
whom we owe the duty of care.

About The Authors

An Obstetrician and Gynecologist in KK Women's Hospital and writer, **Dr Tan Thiam Chye** co-authors the internationally best-selling "Practical O&G Handbook for the General Practitioner". Being a proponent of medical education, he is a faculty teacher in Duke-NUS Graduate Medical School and co-ordinates the OBGYN curriculum since 2007. He takes charge of OBGYN junior doctors' training and education programmes since 2004. A regular newspaper and magazine advice columnist, he also frequently gives public talks on women's health issues. Dr Tan contributed the chapter "Code Green" to the best-selling "Chicken Soup for the Singapore Soul."

Dr Tan Kim Teng (commonly known as KT Tan to her patients) is a senior consultant in KK Women's and Children's Hospital. She is the Head of the Department of General Obstetrics and Gynecology since 2005. She runs a busy clinical practice in both obstetrics and gynecology. She is also the co-author of the internationally best-selling Practical O&G Handbook for the General Practitioner (2006).

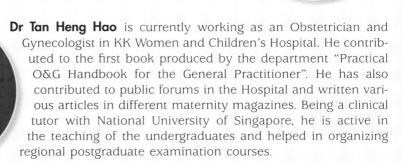

Dr Tan Heng Hao is currently working as an Obstetrician and Gynecologist in KK Women and Children's Hospital. He contributed to the first book produced by the department "Practical O&G Handbook for the General Practitioner". He has also contributed to public forums in the Hospital and written various articles in different maternity magazines. Being a clinical tutor with National University of Singapore, he is active in the teaching of the undergraduates and helped in organizing regional postgraduate examination courses.

Clinical Associate Professor John Tee Chee Seng is a senior consultant obstetrician and gynecologist with KK Women's and Children's Hospital and has been working there since 1989. He was the former Head of Department of General Obstetrics and Gynecology from 1999 till 2004 and the Division Chairman of Obstetrics and Gynecology since 2005. He has special interest in prenatal screening, diagnosis of fetal abnormality as well as fetal surveillance during labor. He is also the OBGYN Clerkship Leader in Duke-NUS Graduate Medical School since 2007.

About KK Women's and Children's Hospital (KKH)

As the largest maternity facility in Singapore, and one of the largest in Southeast Asia, KKH provides care for about 12,000 women and their babies every year. This amounts to about one-third of the total number of babies born in Singapore.

As a leading hospital and international tertiary referral center for women and children, KKH constantly strives to achieve a higher standard in clinical care. KKH is the first hospital in the Asia Pacific to receive the prestigious Asian Hospital Management Award (AHMA) in 2004, for measures taken to improve the safety of women in labor and their newborns. KKH has gained accreditation from the US-based Joint Commission International (JCI) in 2005, which affirmed the quality of our patient care and safety. This is a first for a Women's and Children's Hospital outside United States. KKH is also the accredited center with the Royal College of Obstetrics & Gynecology (United Kingdom), the International Society for Ultrasound in Obstetrics and Gynecology and the Fetal Medicine Foundation, for obstetric ultrasound scans.

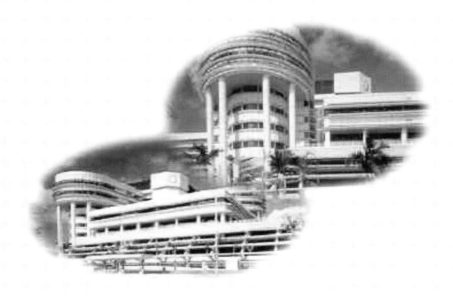

The hospital is recognized for its integrated labor ward risk management program, a comprehensive risk management program that features speedy staff mobilization, constant reviews and audits, training as well as a computerized early-warning system. The program identifies and manages potential risks in the delivery suite, thus helping to improve the safety of women in labor and their newborns. So successful is the program in ensuring patient safety that KKH's perinatal mortality rate for 2005 is 4.9 per 1,000 births — one of the lowest in the world. The average time of delivering a baby in a Crash Cesarean Section for dire emergencies is as low as 7.6 minutes!

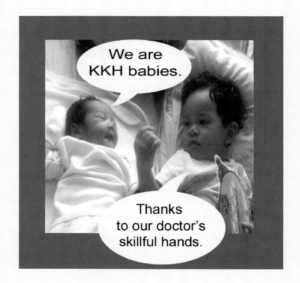

KK Women's and Children's Hospital was also awarded the ISO 9000, ISO 14000 and OH-SAS 18000 certification in 2007.

In addition, the Vermont Oxford Network data shows that standard of baby care in KKH Neonatal Intensive Care Unit is high and among the best in the world.

Book Reviews

"**The New Art and Science of Pregnancy and Childbirth** is very well written by experienced obstetricians who together have many decades of collective experience in the care of thousands of women through their pregnancies. They are clearly cognisant of all the fears and anxieties that every pregnant woman faces and the answers to these are found in the pages of this book. I'm sure this book will help make this special period in a woman's life even more enjoyable. I would highly recommend this book to all women."

Professor Ivy Ng
Chief Executive Officer, KK Women's and Children's Hospital
Senior Consultant Pediatrician

"**The New Art and Science of Pregnancy and Childbirth** demystifies the myriad of queries, concerns, worries and myths related to pregnancy from the stage of planning for pregnancy, through the course of pregnancy and delivery into the postnatal period. The information is expertly presented in a clear and concise manner, from a local perspective, allowing couples to obtain a realistic expectation of how their pregnancy will progress. The book is well organised such that it can either be easily read from cover to cover or by targeting the specific chapters of interest, all of which are well cross-referenced. The breath and depth of coverage of the varied pregnancy-related issues impresses upon me the immense cumulative expertise, which has been gleaned by the authors and their contributors through their years of experience. This book truly does tell you 'What you want to know from your obstetrician'. I have no doubt that couples that are either currently pregnant or planning a pregnancy will find this book extremely useful and interesting."

Dr Kenneth Kwek Yung Chiang
Senior Consultant Obstetrician and Gynecologist, KK Women's and Children's Hospital
Head, Department of Maternal Fetal Medicine and Peripartum Unit
Facility Director, Singapore Cord Blood Banking
Co-chair, KKH Research Committee

Acknowledgements

PRINCIPAL CONTRIBUTORS
FROM KK WOMEN'S AND CHILDREN'S HOSPITAL

This book would not have been possible without the invaluable contributions from our colleagues.

Clinical Associate Professor Tan Kok Hian
Senior Consultant Obstetrician and Gynecologist
Head, Perinatal Audit & Epidemiology, Department of Maternal Fetal Medicine
Director, Clinical Quality
Deputy Chairman, Division of Obstetrics and Gynecology

Clinical Associate Professor George SH Yeo
Chief of Obstetrics
Senior Consultant Obstetrician and Gynecologist
Head, Obstetric Ultrasound & Prenatal Diagnosis Unit
Director, KK Antenatal Diagnostic Centre

Dr Lee Lih Charn
Senior Consultant Obstetrician & Gynecologist
Director, Urogynecological Centre

Dr Judy Wong Pui Ling
Consultant Obstetrician and Gynecologist
Deputy Head, Department of General Obstetrics and Gynecology

Dr Wee Horng Yen
Consultant Obstetrician and Gynecologist
Director, KK Women Wellness Center

Dr Goh Shen Li
Obstetrician and Gynecologist

Dr Jasmine Mohd
Obstetrician and Gynecologist

Dr Cynthia Kew
Obstetrician and Gynecologist

Dr Chin Pui See
Obstetrician and Gynecologist

Dr Choey Wei Yen
Obstetrician and Gynecologist

CHAPTER CONTRIBUTORS FROM KK WOMEN'S AND CHILDREN'S HOSPITAL

Dr Helen Chen
Consultant Psychiatrist
Head, Mental Wellness Service
For Chapter on "Baby blues and depression" and Co-contributor for "Pregnancy loss and ways to cope"

Dr Ong Wee Sian
Consultant Sports Physician
Head, Sports Medicine Service
For Chapter on "Exercise in pregnancy"

Dr Khoo Poh Choo
Senior Consultant Neonatologist
Department of Neonatology and Child Development Unit
For Chapters on "Care of the newborn" and "Baby's vaccination"

Dr Eileen Lew
Consultant Anesthetist
Women's Anesthesia
For Chapter on "I want a painless labour"

Ms Christine Ong
Chief Dietitian
For Chapter on "Eating right for breastfeeding"

Ms Phuah Kar Yin
Senior Dietitian
For Chapter on "Nutrition during pregnancy – eating right for two"

Ms Thilagamangai
Nurse Clinician, Delivery Suite
For Chapter on "What should I pack before my due date? What can I expect once I am admitted into the delivery suite?"

Ms Cynthia Pang
Lactation Consultant
For Chapter on "Breastfeeding"

Ms June Chew
Senior Physiotherapist
For Chapter on "Pelvic Floor exercises"

Ms Carol Remedios
Senior Physiotherapist
For Chapter on "Aqua exercise in pregnancy"

Ms Catherine Chua
Senior Physiotherapist
For Chapter on "Returning to pre-pregnancy weight and shape"

Ms Chua Yew Lan
Pharmacist
For Chapter on "Safe medication in pregnancy and breastfeeding"

INVITED GUEST CHAPTER CONTRIBUTORS

Clinical Associate Professor Giam Yoke Chin
Senior Consultant Dermatologist
National Skin Centre
For Chapter on "Skin care in pregnancy"

Dr Marina Teh
Consultant Orthodontist
Pacific Healthcare Specialist Centre
For Chapter on "Dental care in pregnancy"

Dr Teo Cheng Peng
Consultant Hematologist and Medical Director
StemCord Private Limited
For Chapter on "Cord blood banking"

Physician Zhong Xi Ming
Eu Yan Sang TCM Centre for Reproductive Health
For Chapters on "Traditional Chinese Medicine (TCM) and pregnancy" and "Traditional Chinese Medicine (TCM) and confinement"

SPONSORSHIP

Bayer Schering Pharma

Dumex

StemCord Private Limited

Wyeth Consumer Healthcare

SPECIAL THANKS

Dr Chin Pui See (Illustrations)

Ms Julieanna Md Noor (Secretariat)

Ms Ong Phei Hong (Secretariat)

Contents

Part 1 : Pre-pregnancy Care

Part 2 : All About Your Pregnancy

Part 3 : Concerns About Your Delivery

Part 4 : Postnatal And Baby Care

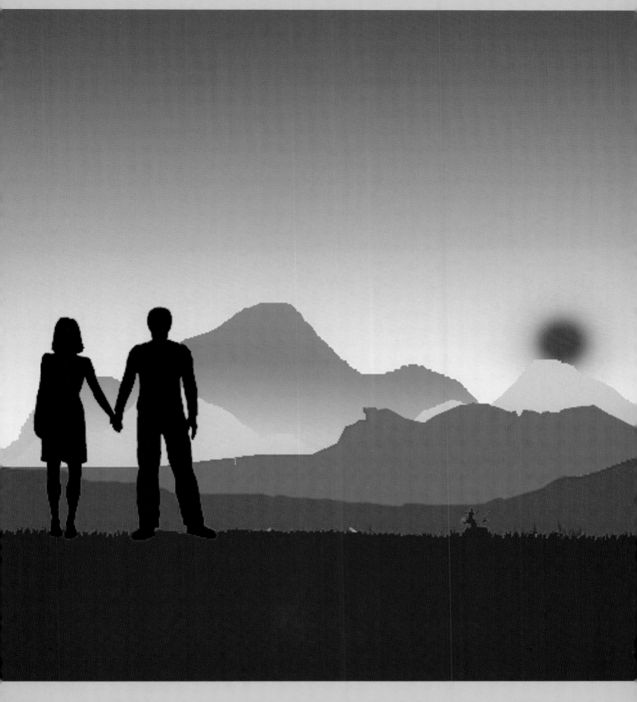

ORE PREGNANCY CARE

Chapter 1
Pre-Pregnancy Preparation

> *Before you were conceived, I wanted you.*
> *Before you were born, I loved you.*
> *Before you were here an hour, I would die for you.*
> *This is the miracle of Mother's love.*
>
> **Maureen Hawkins**

Pregnancy is an exciting and rewarding experience for any woman. Pre-pregnancy preparation is essential in the journey of pregnancy. Being well prepared would optimize your chance of a smooth pregnancy and healthy baby. It prepares you both physically and emotionally.

Now that you have decided to embark on the journey of motherhood, let us see how you can prepare yourself for a healthy pregnancy. Ideally, you should start at least three months before you conceive, but it is never too late either.

Start Young

The prime of your fertility is when you are 20–24 years old, with a sharp decline from 35 years old onwards. On average, there is a drop of 3% in fertility with each increasing year of the woman's age (Figure 1.1). The chance of genetic abnormalities like Down syndrome as well as complications in pregnancy like miscarriages, high blood pressure and diabetes, increase as you grow older, particularly beyond 35 years of age. So, start young when you are in your prime!

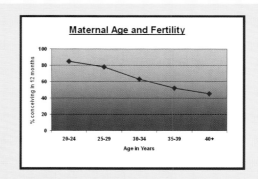

Figure 1.1 Pregnancy rate and mother's age.

Pre-pregnancy Supplementation

It is important to take a diet balanced in calories, carbohydrates, proteins and fibers. Folic acid is a type of vitamin B that is needed for the formation of blood cells and the development of baby's nervous system. It has been shown to reduce the chance of a baby having neural tube defects (spinal cord and brain abnormalities) (Figure 1.2). A simple way is to take a folic acid supplement of 5 mg at least three months before conception and continue for the first 12 weeks of pregnancy.

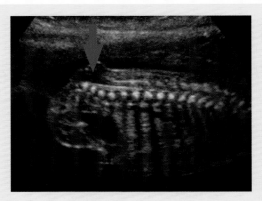

Figure 1.2 Defect at lower spine (arrow).

Pre-conception Check-up

Visit a gynecologist to discuss your chance of conception, previous medical problems that may affect your pregnancy, family history of genetic problems and immunization history. Your check-up may include a PAP smear test, thalassemia (genetic blood disorder) test and rubella (German measles) screening. A pelvic ultrasound scan can also be performed to check for ovarian cysts or fibroids in the womb.

Optimize Your Medical Conditions

Controlling your medical conditions such as diabetes mellitus and hypertension improves the prognosis for you and your baby. Consult your obstetrician early as pregnancy could be complicated with such medical conditions. If the medical conditions are well-controlled before you conceive, you are more likely to have a smooth pregnancy and a healthy baby.

Other existing medical conditions that could affect or be affected by pregnancy include:

- Auto-immune diseases such as systemic lupus erythematosus and rheumatoid arthritis
- Epilepsy
- Thyroid disorders
- Asthma
- Anemia such as iron-deficiency anemia or thalassemia

- Kidney disease
- Heart disease
- Deep vein thrombosis or pulmonary embolism (blood clots in legs or lungs)
- Depression

It is possible to have a successful pregnancy if you have one of these chronic conditions, but it may be considered a *high risk pregnancy* and you will have to take some special precautions.

If you are on chronic medication for these conditions, your gynecologist will want to assess them in terms of their effect on you and your developing baby. For example, if you are a known diabetic on oral medication, you will need to change to insulin injections once your pregnancy is confirmed.

Avoid High-risk Activities

It is advisable to stop smoking. Substance abuse and smoking are associated with miscarriages, slowing of baby's growth in the womb, pre-mature delivery and bleeding in the placenta. Avoid excessive alcohol and binge drinking. This can lead to congenital malformations and mental impairment of your baby.

FREQUENTLY ASKED QUESTIONS

What are some problems that older mothers may face during pregnancy?

It is important to reiterate that most pregnancies in older mothers **have a good outcome**. Traditionally, an older mother is defined as any expectant mother who is 35 years old or more at her expected date of delivery.

There is an increased incidence of chromosomal problems as the quality of the egg may deteriorate with advancing maternal age. In particular, there is an increased risk of Down's Syndrome when compared to a younger age group. There is also an increased risk of twin pregnancy (see Chapter 22). In addition, older mothers have an increased risk of miscarriages.

Overall, there is an increased tendency to medical conditions such as pregnancy-induced hypertension and gestational diabetes. It is important for any mother with an advanced maternal age to see an obstetrician early so that proper follow-up and tests can be performed.

Chapter 2
Pre-Pregnancy Vaccination

Screening for Vaccine-Preventable Diseases

Before you conceive, it is advisable to get yourself screened for vaccine-preventable illnesses. Should you contract any of these diseases during pregnancy, they could have a serious impact on you and your baby's wellbeing.

These diseases include:

- Rubella (German measles)
- Varicella (Chicken pox)
- Hepatitis B

Once you are up to date with your vaccinations, you can proceed with your plans to conceive.

IMPORTANT!

Get yourself vaccinated at least three months before pregnancy if you are not immunized against these diseases.

Rubella (German Measles)

Rubella is very contagious. It spreads when you breathe in droplets of respiratory secretions exhaled by an infected person. The *Rubella* virus causes fever and a rash that starts on the face and spreads to the body, and then to the arms and legs.

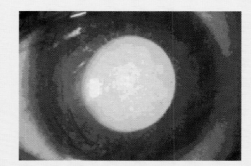

Figure 2.1 Congenital Rubella Syndrome causes cataract and blindness in the affected baby.

Rubella is not serious in children, but it can become very serious to fetuses, especially in the first four months of pregnancy. The risk of the mother passing the infection to the baby can be up to 90% in the first trimester (first 12 weeks of pregnancy). Heart damage, blindness, deafness and mental retardation may develop in the baby (Figure 2.1). The mother can also have a miscarriage or even a stillbirth.

Fortunately, rubella is no longer common because most babies are immunized against it as part of the MMR (measles, mumps, rubella) vaccine when they are 12 months old.

Varicella zoster (Chicken Pox) Infection

Like rubella, chicken pox is very infectious. As with the rubella virus, the *Herpes zoster* virus spreads when you inhale droplets of respiratory secretions exhaled by an infected person.

A non-immunized person may catch chicken pox by being in the same room with an infected person. Symptoms may not appear until ten days to three weeks after infection. The patient often has fever and lethargy, followed by an itchy rash of watery blisters. The blisters will burst after a week and form crusts before healing.

Chicken pox is uncommon in pregnancy. If it does occur in pregnancy, most women and baby suffer no serious effects. However, in 1–2 out of every 100 cases, the baby may be affected by skin blisters, scarring or even organ damage, especially in the first five months of pregnancy. These abnormalities may not be detected with ultrasound scans during pregnancy. They may only be diagnosed after the baby is delivered. Some pregnant women may also develop serious forms of infection in the chest or brain.

If the baby is born within seven days of the mother developing chicken pox, he/she may get a very severe form of the illness.

All it takes is a simple blood test to check if you are immune to the chicken pox virus. If you are not immune, get yourself vaccinated before you conceive.

Hepatitis B

Hepatitis B is a liver infection caused by *Hepatitis B* viruses. The infection can be acute or chronic. Most chronic carriers have no symptoms. You can become infected by Hepatitis B through sexual contact or by exposure to infected body fluids such as saliva.

If you are a chronic carrier of Hepatitis B, you can pass the infection to your baby. Infected infants do not appear to be at a higher risk of birth defects.

However, they have a 25% chance of dying from liver-related diseases such as chronic hepatitis, cirrhosis, and liver cancer later in life.

To prevent the baby from being infected, he/she should be vaccinated with an injection of the Hepatitis B vaccine and anti-bodies **immediately** after delivery. Once the baby is vaccinated against Hepatitis B, the mother can continue to breastfeed even if she is a carrier.

FREQUENTLY ASKED QUESTIONS

1. Does vaccination carry any risks for the developing fetus?

There is no evidence that vaccinating pregnant women poses any risk to the developing fetus. The pregnant woman may be vaccinated with "killed" (inactivated) viruses, bacterial vaccines or toxoids. Examples of "killed" vaccines are flu, Hepatitis B and tetanus vaccines.

We recommend that you avoid "live" virus vaccines (like measles, mumps, and rubella) that contain small parts of the actual virus. They may cause miscarriage or birth defects if they are transmitted to the baby. This risk is very small though.

Other examples of "live" virus vaccines include chicken pox, smallpox, Bacillus Calmette-Guerin (BCG) and poliomyelitis vaccines.

2. Once I get a "live" virus vaccination, how long do I need to wait to attempt to conceive?

If you receive a "live" virus vaccine, you need to wait at least three months before you try to conceive. Your body will need time to flush out the injected viruses.

However, if you become pregnant accidentally before the three months' period, do not be alarmed. Consult your obstetrician immediately. The risk of your baby being affected is very small and you may not need to terminate the pregnancy.

3. Can I get other childhood diseases again?

Chicken pox, German measles and mumps generally give you a lifelong immunity once you have had them. If you are unsure of your immunity status, consult your obstetrician to do a simple blood test.

4. Is it safe for me to get a flu vaccine during pregnancy?

Getting the flu while pregnant may lead to complications in some women. These include high fever and lung infections, which may require hospitalization. It has also been suggested that flu may increase the rate of miscarriage. The flu vaccine can be **safely** administered to pregnant women to prevent these complications, especially during the flu season.

5. **I seem to get more colds and flu than usual since my pregnancy began. Why is this so?**
Pregnant women tend to get more colds and flu due to the weakened immune system during pregnancy. The body has to lower its defenses to make sure that the baby is not rejected. Unfortunately, pregnant women then become more susceptible to minor flu and colds than before.

6. **Which travel vaccine is safe and recommended for pregnancy?**
You can consider meningococcal and rabies vaccine if these diseases are endemic in the country which you are traveling to. The safety of vaccines for yellow fever, Hepatitis A and typhoid is *not yet established* in pregnancy.

7. **Are vaccinations safe for breastfeeding?**
Be rest assured that *vaccinations are safe for breastfeeding* for both the "live" as well as inactivated vaccines.

Chapter 3

Sexual Positions and Timing of Conception

> A great joy is coming.
>
> **Anonymous**

Sexual relation is an integral aspect of any healthy marriage. It is important that both partners are comfortable and enjoy the intimacy. However, patients often ask, "Doc, what is the best sexual position to adopt for conception?"

Let us examine the different sexual positions and determine their varying degrees of effectiveness.

Missionary Position

Many experts believe that the missionary position (man on top) affords the best opportunity for baby-making. This position allows for the deepest penetration and as a result, places the sperms closer to the cervix.

For additional effectiveness, the woman can try elevating her hips with a pillow so that her cervix is exposed to the maximum amount of semen.

Rear Entry

Rear entry, when the man enters the woman from behind, either lying down or kneeling, can also deposit the sperms close to the cervix to aid conception.

Side Entry

Lying side-by-side can be a relaxing position and easier on a partner who is overweight or has chronic back problems.

Effective Maneuvres

A woman can further in-
crease the likelihood of
conception by remaining in
bed for up to half an hour
following intercourse, preferably on her back and with
a pillow under her pelvic
region. In theory, this provides the sperms with additional travel time up to the
fallopian tube with the aid
of gravity.

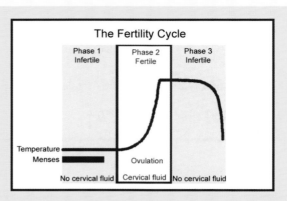

Figure 3.1 Basal body temperature and cervical
mucus to predict ovulation.

The contractions that
accompany a female's orgasm may help carry the sperms further into the
cervix.

Sexual Positions that are not Recommended for Conception

Avoid having sex while sitting, standing or with female partner on top.
These positions defy gravity and may discourage the upward mobility of the
sperms.

Predicting Your Timing of Ovulation

You can increase your chances of getting pregnant by timing your sexual intercourse close to your time of ovulation (releasing of your egg).

However, keep in mind that every woman's menstrual cycle is different.
Normal cycles can vary from 21 days to 35 days. We use the 28-day cycle as
an average. There are several ways to predict ovulation.

1. Basal body temperature

You will experience a slight increase in your body temperature just *after* ovulation. Measure your body temperature every morning after waking up and keep
a record of your body temperature every day. After a few cycles, a pattern
should emerge (Figure 3.1).

2. Changes in your body

Be vigilant of changes in your body. The cervical mucus is noted to be thin-
ner and clearer during ovulation. Another indication of ovulation is mild lower

tummy pain during mid-cycle when the egg is released from the follicle in the ovary. This is called *mittelschmerz*, and is sometimes accompanied by mid-cycle spotting or mild bleeding.

3. Ovulation test kits

There are test kits to predict ovulation which are easy to use. The test strip is placed under a stream of urine when the woman first wakes up in the morning. The strip changes color to indicate hormonal changes related to ovulation. These kits are fairly accurate.

However, the most important factor is to have regular sexual intercourse. We suggest **having sex at least three times a week** if you are trying to conceive.

For women with regular 28-day menstrual cycles, your most fertile period is between Day 11 to Day 18 of your last menstrual period. And, remember, the ovulated egg only lives from 24–48 hours, sperms live for 72 hours!

Chapter 4

Baby Gender Selection — Boy or Girl?

> *Children enhance you.*
>
> **Melanie Griffith**

There is now a great deal of interest generated over this topic. Proponents of gender selection believe that it gives the couple a choice in choosing their child's gender. Opponents question the morality of such a practice.

Gender selection is **not allowed** in Assisted Reproductive Techinques in Singapore. In this chapter, we will discuss some of the natural gender selection techniques that have been put forward. **However, it must be noted that these methods are not scientifically proven**.

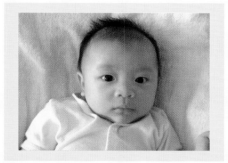

How is Your Baby's Sex Determined?

A baby is conceived from the fertilization of a sperm and an egg. The egg can only carry an X chromosome while a sperm can possess either a X or Y chromosome from the father. If an X-carrying sperm fertilizes the egg, a baby girl (XX) will be conceived. If a Y-carrying sperm fertilizes the egg, a baby boy (XY) will be

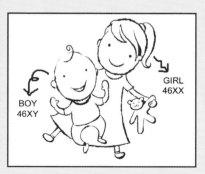

Figure 4.1 Gender and karyotype (genetic makeup).

conceived. Therefore, it is evident that the **father 'influences' the gender of his offspring**.

Scientific Basis for Gender Selection

One of the theories suggested is that the sperm with the Y chromosome, known as the androsperm (resulting in a male offspring), is tiny and fragile but moves very quickly. On the contrary, the sperm with the X chromosome, known as the gynosperm (resulting in a female offspring), is larger and hardier with a longer lifespan, but moves rather sluggishly.

Therefore, the male sperm would race to meet the egg much faster than the female sperm. But they have a shorter lifespan and would not be able to survive in an acidic vaginal environment.

Gender Selection Options — Natural Methods

1. Shettles method (male offspring)

Time the intercourse to as close to the ovulation as possible — preferably within 24 hours before ovulation. There should be a period of abstinence of about 3–4 days in order to maximize the number of male sperms produced.

Penetration at the moment of ejaculation should be as deep as possible, e.g. via rear entry. This ensures that the sperms are deposited above the neck of the cervix, where the vaginal environment is more alkaline and thus, more favorable for the male sperms to survive. This increases the chances of the male sperms reaching the egg faster than the female sperms.

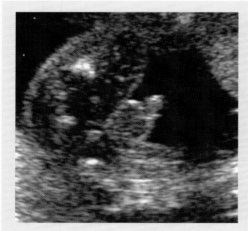 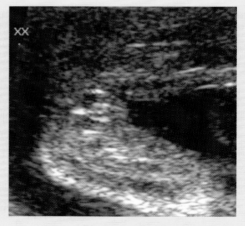

Figure 4.2 Ultrasound picture showing a baby boy.   Figure 4.3 Ultrasound picture showing a baby girl.

2. *Shettles method (female offspring)*

The converse to the above-mentioned will hold true. Timing the intercourse two days prior to ovulation will ensure that only the female sperms will survive till fertilization.

Shallow penetration, e.g. man-on-top will ensure that the sperms are deposited at the mouth of the cervix. This favors the survival of the female sperms. Some have advocated avoiding a female orgasm as this keeps the vaginal environment highly acidic.

Gender Selection Kits

Many of such kits are now available and can be found on the Internet. However, they can be costly. They aim to help guide the couples choose the gender of their child over one ovulatory cycle, by following the instructions attached. Most are based on the Shettles method and comprise of various ovulation predictor test sticks aided by application of a vaginal douche to help make the environment more suitable for either a male or female sperm.

Myths

As in all things, various myths do exist and have no scientific basis at all, other than being handed down from generations within the family. They include a whole host of things such as the choice of diet, sleeping positions, having intercourse on certain calendar days and for either of the partner to reach an orgasm first. These are useless with regards to gender selection and should be read only purely for the sake of interest.

Chapter 5

I Can't Get Pregnant!
Is There Anything Wrong?

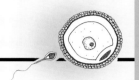

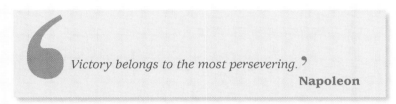

> *Victory belongs to the most persevering.*
> **Napoleon**

How Does a Pregnancy Happen?

Conception can only happen when a sperm swims up into the womb before fertilizing an egg in the fallopian tube. This allows the fertilized embryo to implant or embed itself into the womb lining, where it will grow into a fetus.

Am I Subfertile?

There is indeed a possibility that something is wrong in you or your partner if you are still not pregnant after a period of trying to conceive. An average couple in their 30s will conceive after about 6 months of trying to do so. Certainly, **any couple that fails to conceive after a year of trying, should seek prompt medical attention**, so that the appropriate investigations and treatment can be carried out.

In our current climate of a hectic schedule, it is important to note that regular sexual intercourse of 2–3 times per week should be happening between the couple before they can be labeled as subfertile. **The most fertile period is usually two weeks before the onset of a women's period if she has a regular cycle**. This is when the egg is released from the ovary into the fallopian tubes.

What can Possibly be Wrong?

It is important to remember that **subfertility is never the fault of any one individual**. There are varying factors that could contribute to a couple not being able to conceive. For a start, one must exclude male or female sexual dysfunction, whereby the sexual act is never carried out anyway. This can lead to a breakdown of the relationship in the long run. There can be many reasons for male sexual dysfunction and an inability to ejaculate. They include impotence, erectile dysfunction, diabetes, prostate surgery or chronic usage of medications, e.g. anti-hypertensives. In the female, vaginismus or pain during sexual intercourse is perhaps the most common cause of female sexual dysfunction.

Various tests may be carried out to further investigate underlying causes. They include:

- A sperm analysis to look out for any sperm abnormalities.
- Hormonal blood tests to confirm ovulation.
- Radiographic tests such as a pelvic ultrasound scan to assess for womb problems or growths. A hystero-salpingogram, that involves the X-ray of

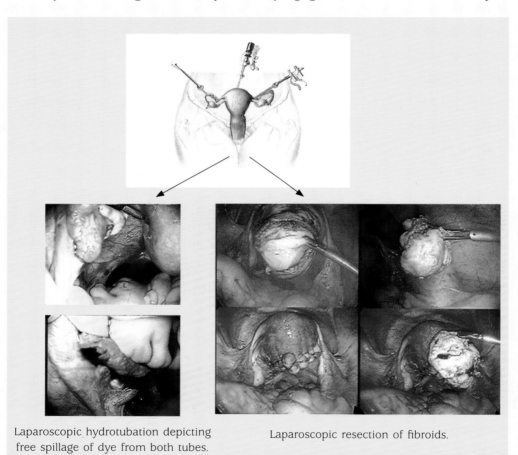

Laparoscopic hydrotubation depicting free spillage of dye from both tubes.

Laparoscopic resection of fibroids.

Figure 5.1 Laparoscopic surgery.

the pelvis after passing of a dye contrast into the womb to assess the patency of the fallopian tubes, can also be performed.

- A key-hole surgical survey of the womb cavity (via hysteroscopy) and the fallopian tubes (via laparoscopy) can also be performed and any gynecological problems may be treated at the same time.

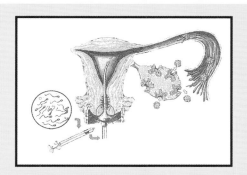

Figure 5.2 Assisted reproductive technique.

In 20% of couples, no identifiable causes can be found (*idiopathic subfertility*). In such cases, treatment is only empirical and assisted reproductive techniques (ARTs) such as intra-uterine insemination or in-vitro fertilization (test-tube baby) can be employed to help the couple conceive. In the remaining 80%, problems can be divided into female factors, male factors or a combination of both.

Female Factor Subfertility

In the female, any factor that prevents the sperm from reaching the egg (ovum) in the fallopian tube will result in subfertility (refer to Figure 5.3).

Anovulation (failure of the ovaries to produce an egg) — This commonly results from stress, excessive weight loss or exercise, poor nutrition, chronic medical conditions, inherent ovarian problems such as polycystic ovarian syndrome or previous ovarian surgeries. They usually manifest as an absence, delay or irregularity in the menses.

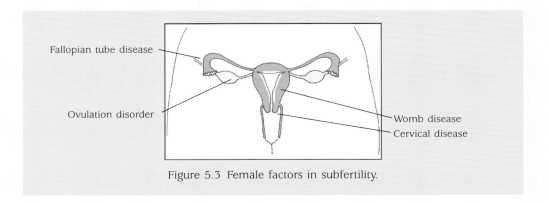

Figure 5.3 Female factors in subfertility.

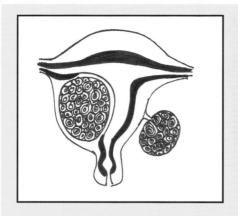 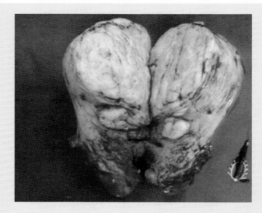

Figure 5.4 Fibroids.

Fallopian tube blockage — Even if an egg is released, blocked fallopian tubes can still prevent fertilization from happening. These may result from previous genital infections, tubal surgeries, endometriosis or pelvic adhesions.

Womb or cervical mucus defects or abnormalities — These can prevent fertilization or implantation, resulting in subfertility. Large fibroids, especially those disrupting the womb cavity, have been known to be associated with an inability to conceive. Womb adhesions (Asherman syndrome) resulting from previous surgeries or instrumentations will result in the obliteration of the entire cavity and prevent subsequent conception. Congenital defects such as septum or abnormal womb structure can contribute to this problem as well.

Endometriosis — This is a very common gynecological condition amongst women in the reproductive age group. It is characterized by the implantation of the womb lining tissue in the abdomen or the pelvic cavity. Menstrual pain and subfertility are the most common symptoms that can affect these women. In severe cases, it can disrupt the fallopian tubes and cause tubal blockage. However, even mild cases have been known to be associated with subfertility and the surgical removal of these deposits can result in an improvement of the fertility.

Male Factor Subfertility

Abnormal sperm parameters can include a low sperm count (oligospermia), lack of sperm (azoospermia), abnormal sperm shape (teratozospermia) or a lack of sperm motility (asthenospermia). There are many underlying factors that may contribute to the above. Prolonged heat exposure may reduce sperm potency, hence explaining the rationale of avoiding tight under-garments. Various other possible underlying causes of poor sperm quality or low counts include alcoholism, recreational drug abuse, environmental toxins and long-term usage of certain medications. More commonly, problems may exist in the testicles or testicular ducts, and these affect sperm production. The testicular problems include varicocele (engorged blood vessels surrounding the testes), undescended testes (even if successfully treated in infancy), previous testicular infections (such as mumps), previous testicular or hernia operations. Testicle duct blockage affects sperm delivery and this can be due to testicle duct scarring (from previous sexually transmitted infections) or an inherent genital tract abnormality.

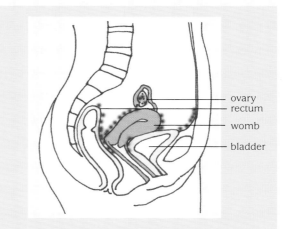

Figure 5.5 Common sites for endometrial growth.

Table 5.1 Analysis of sperm.

Human Sperm Analysis	
Sperm Parameters	*Normal Range (WHO criteria, 1992)*
Volume	≥ 2.0 mL
pH	7.2–8.0
Concentration	≥ 20 x 10^6 spermatozoa/mL
Motility	≥ 50% forward progression
Morphology	≥ 15% normal forms (Kruger strict criteria)
White blood cells	< 1 x 10^6/mL

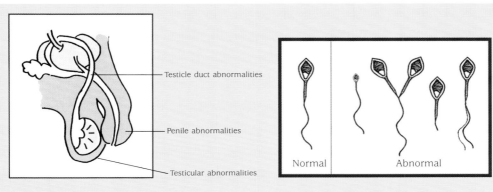

Figure 5.6 Male problems in subfertility.

Figure 5.7 Sperm abnormalities.

FREQUENTLY ASKED QUESTIONS

1. When and why should I seek medical attention if I am unable to conceive?

Any couple who cannot conceive after 12 months of regular sexual intercourse should seek immediate medical attention. It is preferable that both the partners see their doctor together so that the appropriate investigations and counseling can take place.

We **advise women aged 35 years and above** to seek medical attention **urgently** as the treatment success is lower in older women.

2. What can be done for subfertility?

Depending on the underlying causes, varying treatment modalities may be offered. In cases of anovulation, drugs that enhance ovulation e.g. **clomiphene** may be prescribed to help the couple conceive. This can result in **minor side effects** such as nausea and bloatedness, **multiple pregnancies** (5–10% chance of twins) and may increase the **risk of ovarian cancer** in cases of prolonged and unregulated usage. Therefore, **clomiphene is usually prescribed for only six ovulatory cycles**.

Laparoscopic (key-hole) surgical interventions can also be used to treat tubal blockages, uterine abnormalities, fibroids or endometriosis.

Assisted reproductive techniques (ARTs), such as intra-uterine inseminations or in-vitro fertilizations (test tube babies), may be employed by reproductive specialists in certain cases. In cases of severe male factor, intra-cytoplasmic sperm injection (ICSI) can be used. This refers to the injection of a single sperm to fertilize the egg. All these can only happen after detailed counseling of the procedural risks and benefits.

In the most extreme cases or for those adverse to assisted reproductive programmes, child adoption can even be considered as a last resort.

Chapter 6

Am I Pregnant?

> *Whether your pregnancy was meticulously planned, medically coaxed, or happened by surprise, one thing is certain — your life will never be the same.*
>
> **Catherine Jones**

You may suspect that you are pregnant when you have unusual symptoms of pregnancy or if you have missed your period. If you have regular periods and have missed your period by a week, it is likely that you are pregnant. However, if you have irregular menstrual cycles, look out for other symptoms of pregnancy (see Chapter 20).

For a start, confirm your suspicion by buying an over-the-counter urine pregnancy test kit. There are many brands of pregnancy test kits available in the market, which are quite reliable. These are available at our local pharmacies. Alternatively, you could go to your doctor for a test.

What is a Pregnancy Test Kit?

During pregnancy, a hormone called human chorionic gonadotrophin (hCG) is produced, which circulates in the blood and is also present in the urine.

The pregnancy test kit detects the presence of hCG in your urine. It is a qualitative test. Some pregnancy test kits are more sensitive than the others but most will be

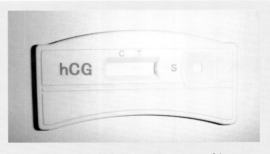

Figure 6.1 Urine pregnancy test kit.

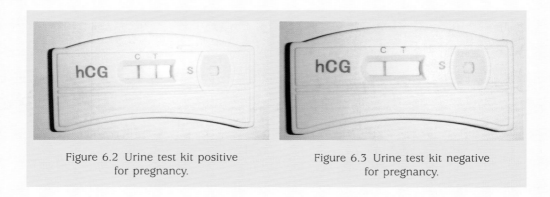

Figure 6.2 Urine test kit positive for pregnancy.

Figure 6.3 Urine test kit negative for pregnancy.

able to detect hCG between the fourth to fifth week of your pregnancy. This means that for those with regular cycles, the test should be positive once you have missed your period by a few days.

Although almost all over-the counter pregnancy test kits detect pregnancy by measuring hCG in the urine, you have to read the instructions for the test kit because instructions for usage are different for different test kits (Figure 6.1).

An indicator will show if you are pregnant. For example, some kits will show two bold lines if positive (Figure 6.2) and one bold line (Figure 6.3) if negative. These indicators are different for various kits.

How Accurate are the Pregnancy Test Kits?

Pregnancy tests are rarely wrong. It is more than 99% accurate. Thus, if your test is negative, it means that you are not pregnant; However, if you are very early in your pregnancy and the test is done too early, there could be insufficient amount of hCG in the urine for the test to detect.

So, if a test comes back negative but you strongly suspect that you are pregnant, repeat the test in a few days' time.

There are rare examples when the hCG level is raised transiently and then drops to zero. This is known as "**biochemical pregnancy**" and could be the cause of a false positive result of the test kit. This initial rise of hCG levels would soon drop in "biochemical pregnancy" and result in a negative test result. Vaginal bleeding occurs soon after, which would coincide with "delayed menses". Also rarely, there could be **occasional ovarian tumors** which secrete hCG and the **false positive result** could be wrongly interpreted as a pregnancy.

FREQUENTLY ASKED QUESTIONS

1. Do I have to test with first morning urine?
Although you can test any time of the day, your first morning urine specimen is usually the most concentrated of the day and would have the most pregnancy hormones in it.

2. When should I take the test if I suspect that I am pregnant?
You can test your urine as early as six days past ovulation but the first day of your missed period is recommended for greatest accuracy.

3. Do I need a blood test for hCG to confirm my pregnancy?
Blood tests for hCG are more accurate in detecting HCG and they can also measure the actual levels of the hormone. These tests may be useful to differentiate a miscarriage when the blood hCG will drop with time or a healthy pregnancy when the blood hCG level will double every two days. Occasionally, we need to follow-up the hCG levels to help us diagnose an early ectopic pregnancy (pregnancy that is outside the womb), which could be potentially life-threatening or confirm a miscarriage.

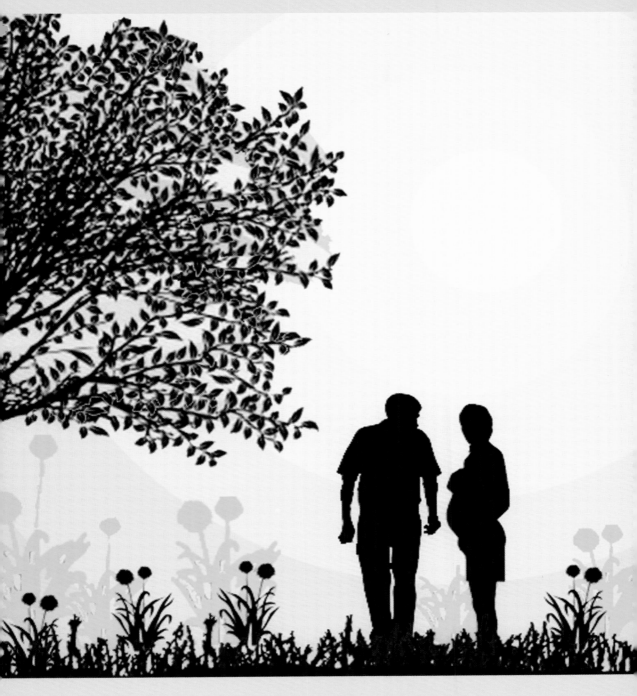

All About Your Pregnancy

Chapter 7

Before the First Antenatal Visit

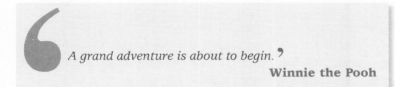

A grand adventure is about to begin.

Winnie the Pooh

After confirming your pregnancy with a self-test kit, what should you do next? Very often, many women find themselves at a loss and do not know what else to do before seeing their obstetricians.

Start Folic Acid Supplementation

Firstly, start supplementation of folic acid (5 mg a day). It is important to note that folic acid is recommended in the first 12 weeks of pregnancy to reduce the risks of spinal cord abnormalities. You can buy these tablets over the counter without a prescription and before your appointment with your doctor.

No Raw Sushi Please

Avoid eating raw food or unprocessed dairy products to prevent gastrointestinal infections, which may affect your baby.

Keep Your Exercise Regime to a Moderate Pace

Exercise is safe in pregnancy. However, not all forms of exercise is appropriate. Swimming and walking are very safe. Generally, avoid exercises that require sudden changes in posture and excessive weight bearing such as squash, tennis and brisk jogging. (For more advice, see Chapter 15 on *"Do's and Don'ts in Pregnancy"*.)

Choosing Your Obstetrician

How would you go about choosing your obstetrician who would diligently look after you in the next 10 months and deliver your baby safely?

Most women will ask their friends, colleagues or relatives for recommendations. Others prefer to be delivered by their own obstetricians who had attended to their previous pregnancies.

These recommendations are important as a reference but obviously, just as "beauty is in the eyes of the beholder", what is great choice for one may not be the same for another!

Delivering in a Restructured Maternity Hospital

In a restructured maternity hospital like **KK Women's and Children's Hospital**, there are specialists on duty round the clock to attend to any problems that you may encounter in your entire pregnancy. Consultation, blood tests, ultrasound scans and medications are all available at affordable rates.

Private care is also available in the restructured hospital. You will be able to choose your own obstetrician who will look after you throughout the entire pregnancy. Of course, he/she will attend to your delivery as well. Thus, it is more personalized as your obstetrician is familiar with your medical history and condition.

The **greatest advantage of delivering in a restructured hospital** is that there are **in-house specialists, anesthetists and pediatricians round the clock**. They would attend to any emergencies immediately and emergency Cesarean sections can be performed without delay. This ensures optimal outcomes for both mother and baby. In addition, affordable and excellent neonatal intensive care facilities are readily available.

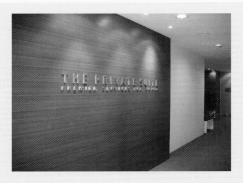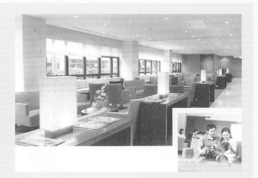

Figure 7.1 The Private Suite in KK Women's and Children's Hospital.

Delivering in a Private Maternity Hospital

Alternatively, you may also choose to be taken care by an obstetrician in a private hospital. The waiting time for your doctor may be shorter. However, the downside is that should you need prolonged hospitalization or if you deliver a premature baby requiring neonatal intensive care, the medical bill can be extremely high.

Be Comfortable with Your Obstetrician and Build a Rapport

You may choose to have your pregnancy followed up in a restructured hospital or in a private clinic. The choice is yours. Do discuss this with your partner.

As the examination and delivery involves examining the most intimate areas, you have to be at ease with your obstetrician. Choose one with whom you have full confidence that your pregnancy will be well managed with the best outcome!

IMPORTANT!

If you experience any persistent pain or bleeding during the pregnancy before your scheduled appointment, you may want to bring forward the appointment date so that an urgent assessment of the pregnancy can be done to exclude miscarriage or an ectopic pregnancy (pregnancy that is outside the womb).

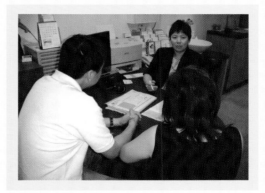

Chapter 8

What Do I Expect During My First Antenatal Visit?

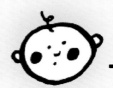

A baby is something you carry inside you for nine months,
in your arms for three years,
and in your heart till the day you die.

Mary Mason

These ten months of antenatal period is a wonderful time for you to enjoy. However, it is crucial that you remain healthy, both physically and emotionally, to enjoy your pregnancy. Antenatal care is part of this preparation and your first visit to your obstetrician after your pregnancy has been confirmed is an important occasion.

Come Prepared

Your obstetrician would love to meet you and your partner together. Come prepared as he/she is likely to enquire about your previous medical history, previous pregnancies and outcomes or family history of genetic syndromes or diabetes. These significant information could impact the outcome of your preg-

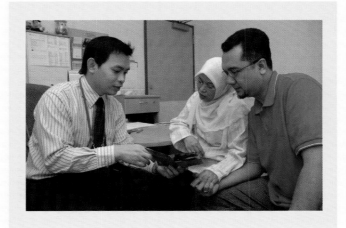

nancy and thus, such pertinent details should not be missed.

Tell Us About Your Lifestyle

If you smoke, drink alcohol, take any regular medication or use recreational drugs, you should inform your obstetrician as these may have an effect on your pregnancy. Rest assured that this information will be kept confidential.

History of Previous Pregnancies

The past obstetric history is crucial in every pregnancy. This includes details of previous miscarriages or abortions (if any), ectopic (outside the womb) pregnancies, any problems with fertility, and any problems during your previous pregnancies or childbirth. If you are unable to recall, try to get hold of the medical summaries of your previous pregnancies.

Record Your Menstrual Calendar

The first thing many mothers-to-be want to know when they first realize that they are pregnant is **WHEN**. When is the baby coming? They would love to know if they are expecting a Christmas baby or one that arrives on an auspicious birth date.

Do keep track of the dates of the first day of your menstrual periods when you are trying to conceive. Many women forget this pertinent detail. The expected date of delivery (EDD) can be calculated from the first day of the last menstrual period (LMP) if you have a regular 28-day menstrual cycle.

Calculate Your EDD

Your baby was conceived about 14 days after the first day of your LMP. **EDD** is at 40 weeks — that is 40 weeks after the first day of your last menstrual

---

EDD calculation using Naegle's rule

Calculate the expected date of delivery (EDD) using Naegle's rule: 280 days from the first day of the last menstrual period (LMP),
i.e. EDD = LMP (first day) + 7 days, and then going forward 9 months

For example: If the LMP is 11/5/2007,
                        EDD = 11 + 7 (day), May + 9 months, i.e. 18/2/2008

(This rule is based on a menstrual cycle of 28 days and assumes ovulation occurred at mid-cycle. Where the cycle is regularly greater than or less than 28 days the calculation has to be adjusted accordingly, e.g. add a further 7 days for a 35 day cycle and subtract a further 7 days for a 21 day cycle.)

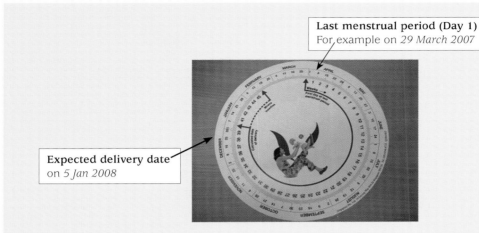

Last menstrual period (Day 1)
For example on *29 March 2007*

Expected delivery date
on *5 Jan 2008*

Figure 8.1 Pregnancy calendar wheel.

period or 280 days after LMP or 38 weeks (or 266 days) since conception. It all corresponds to the same EDD. Amazing, isn't it?

However, your pregnancy is only full-term at 37 weeks after LMP, i.e. your baby is fully matured and ready for delivery at any time. So get your maternity bag and baby cot ready by then!

Preterm (premature) delivery refers to a delivery before 37 completed weeks after LMP.

Use of Pregnancy Calendar Wheel

Most obstetricians are familiar with the pregnancy calender wheel (Figure 8.1). It helps estimate the EDD based on the LMP or dating scan.

Do not be too worried if you have irregular periods or cannot recall your LMP. The most accurate dating is from

DID YOU KNOW?

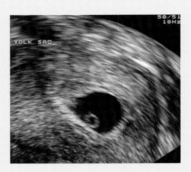

- Your baby's heart can be seen after **6 weeks of LMP**.
- At this stage, the baby's length is now 4 mm. The embryonic period starts and your baby's organs start to form.
- Hair begins to sprout by then.
- Brain waves can also be detected.

first trimester ultrasound measurement of your baby's size. Thus, see your obstetrician early in the first 12 weeks of your pregnancy in order to get an accurate due date.

Pregnancy date calculator from the Internet

There are several pregnancy date calculators that are freely available from the Internet. Do a search engine for "pregnancy date calculator" and you will find them.

FREQUENTLY ASKED QUESTION

I am getting more forgetful and absent-minded since my pregnancy began. Is this normal?

Do not be alarmed if you feel absent-minded and forgetful in pregnancy. You may find yourself misplacing your purse, forgetting to return phone calls, or going off to fetch something only to discover you have forgotten what you are looking for. This is reported by many mothers-to-be.

The exact cause is unknown. Hormonal changes, stress as well as pre-occupation with thoughts of the pregnancy can contribute to this absent-mindedness.

Sleep could also be erratic during your pregnancy. You may become even more forgetful if you are tired during the day.

Chapter 9

Is My Baby Normal?

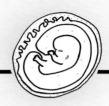

> *Everything grows rounder and wider and weirder,*
> *and I sit here in the middle of it all*
> *and wonder who in the world you will turn out to be.*
> **Carrie Fisher**

After conception and throughout the course of your pregnancy, your baby goes through various phases of growth and development as it implants into the womb and matures into a full term fetus.

Your pregnancy can be generally divided into three main phases:

- **First trimester** — Week 1–12 of pregnancy
- **Second trimester** — Week 13–28 of pregnancy
- **Third trimester** — Week 29–40 of pregnancy

These periods are important as varying stages of fetal development are present in each of the trimesters. The symptoms that you may experience are different. However, this is just a guide and each pregnancy could be different.

First Trimester: Week 1–6

Baby development — This is still considered the **embryonic stage**. It arises just after fertilization of the egg and subsequent implantation of the embryo into the womb lining. The various structures of your baby are not yet fully developed. As the weeks pass:

- The outer layers of the fertilized egg (known as the outer cell mass) will form the eventual placenta
- The inner layers of the fertilized egg (known as the inner cell mass) will give rise to the brain, lungs, central nervous and intestinal systems

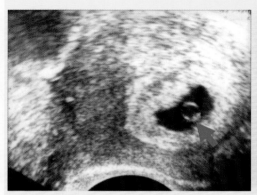 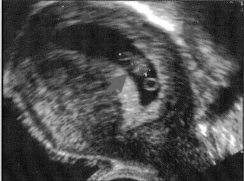

Figure 9.1 Yolk sac at 5 weeks (arrow).   Figure 9.2 Fetus at 6 weeks (arrow).

This is a period whereby the developing organs are highly sensitive to teratogens (drugs affecting the development of baby). Major defects may be produced during this period should there be an exposure to these teratogens. By the end of week 6, the embryo measures about 4–5 mm and the heart starts to beat and can be detected on a scan at the end of this stage.

Your symptoms — You may feel absolutely fine and the first clue to your pregnancy could be the fact that you just **missed your period**. It is crucial that you consult your doctor if you are taking any long term medications.

First Trimester: Week 6–12

Baby development — The baby can now be **considered a fetus** and this stage is a time of rapid growth. The various vital organs are formed as the body straightens. By week 12, most of the major organ systems would have been developed and the baby, known as a fetus, takes on a more recognizable form. It measures about **6 cm** from head to buttocks. The following changes are observed:

- The head is also growing to accommodate the enlarging brain.
- The eyelids are present in the shape of folds and by the end of week 12, they will meet and fuse, remaining closed until the end of month 6.
- The external genitalia are also well differentiated at the end of this stage.
- The limbs continue to develop, and nails appear on the digits. The moving limbs can be visualized but the movements cannot be felt until a few weeks later.

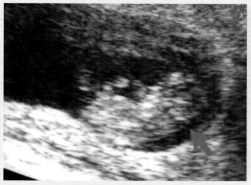

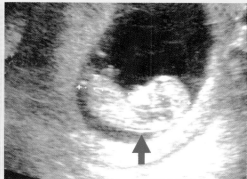

Figure 9.3 Fetus at 9 weeks (arrow).   Figure 9.4 Fetus at 12 weeks (arrow).

After week 16, the baby is less likely to be sensitive to the detrimental effects of teratogens as most of the organs would have developed.

Your symptoms — Your pregnancy hormones will begin to rise by now. You may start to experience the unmistakable early **symptoms of pregnancy** such as **morning sickness, breast tenderness and fatigue**. Your urine pregnancy test will definitely be positive by now.

Second Trimester: Week 13–16

Baby development — The baby continues to grow in size. The proportion of growth is such that the head is still considerably larger than the body. With the continued development of the genitalia, the gender may be discernable by the end of this stage. The limbs are now fully developed and can move vigorously at times.

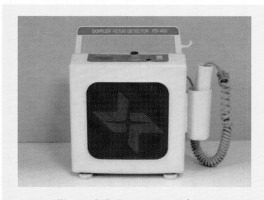

Figure 9.5 Doptone machine.

Your symptoms — By now, the early symptoms would have lessened and your appetite starts to return. Your weight would also begin to increase gradually. Your breasts will continue to enlarge and your nipples will darken.

Your womb would have risen out of your pelvis by now and can be felt on palpation of your abdomen. The baby's heart beat can also be obtained through a doptone machine placed on the womb.

Second Trimester: Week 17–24

Baby development — The baby continues to grow and mature. Hair on the head develops while fine hairs on the body (lanugo) appear.

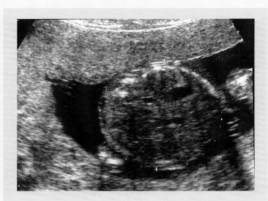

Figure 9.6 Measurement of the fetal abdominal girth at 20 weeks.

Your symptoms — Your physical discomforts of the pregnancy will start to show. They may include the appearance of stretch marks, backaches and a sensation of shortness of breath and palpitations, owing to the enlarging womb. A screening scan should be performed at around 20–22 weeks to exclude any structural abnormalities. You may even begin to feel the baby's movements — known as 'quickening'.

Second Trimester: Week 25–28

Baby development — The eyelids open and the eye lens can be seen. After 24 weeks, the baby is considered by many to be potentially viable. With modern advanced neonatal care, the baby delivered prematurely between 24–28 weeks of pregnancy has a fairly good chance of survival. By the end of 28 weeks, the baby should weigh about 1 kg.

Your symptoms — Your physical discomforts, as described above, will continue to worsen and varicose veins may also begin to appear on your legs. Sleeping at night may start to trouble you. It is important to find your own sleeping position to make yourself comfortable. Having a support for your tummy as you lie on your side to prevent any compression on your major blood vessels may be a good idea.

Third Trimester: Week 29–34

Baby development — The lanugo hairs on the body start to disappear and the skin becomes more pinkish. Fat beneath the skin accumulates and the fetus appears rounder. The fetal movements are more varied now and may alternate between a state of rest and active moving. Babies born after 34 weeks have a very good prognosis.

Your symptoms — Your tummy feels taut and you may begin to feel irregular painless tightenings over your womb. These are also known as 'Braxton-Hicks' contractions and are usually insignificant if there is no associated show or leaking liquor. Your baby becomes considerably heavier and your backache and fatigue may increase.

You may also be experiencing shortness of breath as the enlarging womb presses against your rib cage. At times, the sudden movements of the baby may be painful and the moving limbs may be felt from the surface of your tummy. Contrary to what most mothers think, your baby is actually still very comfortable in the womb despite the increase in size.

Heartburn may increase due to the enlarging womb and reduction in gastric movements. The milk glands in your breasts have started to produce colostrum. This provides nutrition to the baby in the breast milk. At this stage, your breasts may even leak colostrum.

Third Trimester: Week 35–40

Baby development — By now, the baby has fully formed and the head is more proportionate when compared to the size of his body. The lanugo hairs would have completely disappeared and the skin smoothened out.

As the expected due date approaches, the head will begin to descend into the pelvis — a phenomenon known as 'engagement'. The baby's weight continues to increase such that it usually weighs more than 2.5 kg at the time of delivery.

Your symptoms — With the increasing weight of your baby, the aches and pains from the ligament stretch in your pelvis will increase. The lower abdominal aches and urination from the pressure on the bladder can be troubling. From 37 weeks onwards, your baby is considered fully matured (full term) and labor contractions can begin at any time. **However, in 10% of women, preterm labor may happen before 37 weeks**.

Chapter 10

Genetic Syndromes in Family: Is My Baby at Risk?

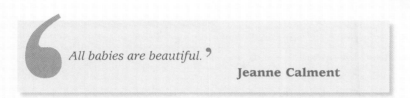

> *All babies are beautiful.*
>
> **Jeanne Calment**

You may be concerned if you have a family history of babies who were born abnormal, or you are worried you might have an unknown genetic problem which may be passed on to your offsprings. Many clues can be gained from keeping family history health records. A genetic counselor may be able to advise you accordingly.

What Causes Genetic Disorders?

Every child inherits 23 pairs of chromosomes from each parent — one from the mum and one from the dad. Each chromosome contains thousands of genes. Genetic disorders can be caused by abnormalities in the number of chromosomes (which are your genetic make up) or a defect in a single gene. In most instances, the genetic disorders are caused by a single gene defect — or what is commonly known as Mendelian genetics. These gene defects may be classified as:

* **Dominant** — one of the genes is defective and over-rides the normal gene, thus

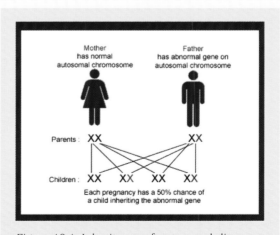

Figure 10.1 Inheritance of autosomal diseases.

the presence of one abnormal gene within the gene pair is adequate for the manifestation of the disease (e.g. polycystic kidney disease, achondroplasia or dwarfism).

- **Recessive** — contrary to the above, the manifestation of the disease requires both genes in the gene pair to be defective (e.g. albinism, cystic fibrosis or thalassemia).

- **Sex-linked** (X-linked) — the defective gene is present in the X chromosome and can be either recessive or dominant. Hence X-linked recessive gene defects tend to manifest in males where the gene is of a XY genotype while X-linked dominant gene defects can manifest in both males (XY) or females (XX) (e.g. hemophilia, muscular dystrophy).

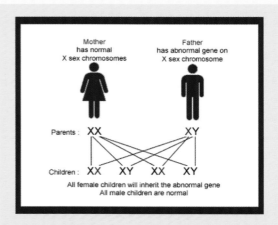

Figure 10.2 Inheritance of sex chromosome linked diseases.

Carriers of recessive defective genes may not have any manifestation and may be unaware. However, if both parents are carriers of the same abnormal gene, there is a 25% chance of having an affected baby for each pregnancy. Carrier testing can be done to determine if you carry one of the two abnormal genes that can cause a specific recessive disorder. Unfortunately, it is not yet possible to test for all genetic conditions.

What is My Risk of Genetic Disease?

In most instances, we are all at a low risk for inherited genetic diseases. However, this risk may increase under certain circumstances. These include a significant family history, ethnicity and heritage. Some genetic syndromes are more common in certain ethnic groups. For instance, 1 in 25 Caucasians of European descent carry the cystic fibrosis mutation gene. Sickle cell trait is more common in Blacks and thalssaemia (an inherited form of anemia) is prevalent in those of Mediterranean or Asian descent.

Do I Need to See a Genetic Counselor?

If you are in any of the following groups, your obstetrician may refer you to see a genetic counselor:

- You had given birth to a genetically abnormal child in your previous pregnancy.
- Your partner is your close relative as the risk of inherited recessive diseases (refer above) increases when the spouses are close relatives, since these defects tend to run within the same family line.
- You have had recurrent pregnancy losses (3 or more consecutive miscarriages).
- You or your partner have blood tests which showed both of you are carriers of a genetic disorder.
- You have a known family history of a serious heritable disorder.
- You have a positive screening test for fetal defect.

How Do Genetic Tests Work?

As these tests carry some risk in the pregnancy, genetic testing will only be conducted if there is a significant chance of the disease manifesting in the baby. A genetic test involves examining a DNA sample from a patient. The DNA sample can come from any human tissue, most commonly from blood samples.

Prenatal diagnostic testing is offered after prenatal screening tests suggest a higher possibility of a genetic disorder, or as a first line diagnostic testing in couples where a specific genetic disorder is present. Prenatal genetic diagnosis provides couples with the option of terminating an affected pregnancy, planning fetal treatment or preparing for the birth of an abnormal child. In general, the test requires a specimen from the fetus, placenta or amniotic fluid for various specific genetic diseases. Other techniques of prenatal genetic diagnosis include radiological studies like MRI, detailed ultrasound of the fetus,

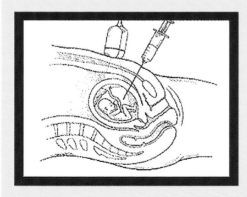

Figure 10.3 Amniocentesis
(from water-bag).

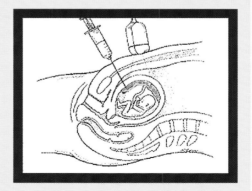

Figure 10.4 Chorionic villous sampling
(from placenta).

and pre-implantation genetic diagnosis in which early embryos created by in-vitro fertilization (test-tube babies) are evaluated to determine the presence of genetic conditions. Unaffected embryos are then selected for implantation into the womb.

Once the sample is obtained, there are several methods of analysis, depending on the type of disorder. For example, chromosomal abnormalities are evaluated by cytogenetic analysis; single gene disorders and inborn errors of metabolism by DNA analysis.

There are many conditions which are amenable to testing in DNA laboratory (thalassaemia, spinal muscular atrophy, fragile X syndrome and myotonic dystrophy), pediatric laboratory (Duchenne Muscular Dystrophy, Hemophilia A) and overseas centers (cystic fibrosis). Let your genetic counselor or obstetrician advise you accordingly.

DID YOU KNOW?

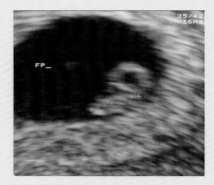

- At **8 weeks gestation,** baby's crown rump length is now 15 mm, about the size of a kidney bean.
- Your baby's genitals start to form, but can only be deciphered clearly on the ultrasound scan after 20 weeks (5 months) gestation.
- The nervous system also starts to coordinate with the muscles so that your baby can now respond to touch.

What are Some of the Issues Relating to Genetic Testing?

It is important to understand that genetic testing is purely voluntary and you should not feel coerced into doing it. The aim of genetic testing is to allow you to predict if you will deliver a normal baby. A negative testing gives you reassurance and a positive result allows you to make informed and deliberate choices with regards to pregnancy continuation or termination (abortion).

There are potential risks of genetic testing. This includes *psychological distress* as the individual faces the prospect of possibly having a hereditary condition and the difficult decision of whether to undergo genetic testing to confirm. Genetic testing may also affect other family members as they may share different views on testing. A positive gene test result may also cause potential genetic discrimination by employers and insurers.

Chapter 11

Down Syndrome Tests

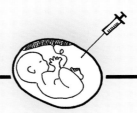

> *The potential possibilities of any child are the most intriguing and stimulating in all creation.*
>
> **Roy L. Wilbur**

What is Down Syndrome?

Down Syndrome is the most common cause of significant mental retardation and learning disability in children. It is caused by a change in chromosomal number (genetic makeup) in the egg before it is fertilized by the sperm (at the time of conception). This usually occurs due to chance, and is more common in older mothers. As a result, the fertilized embryo contains an **extra chromosome 21** making it three instead of the usual pair (hence the name trisomy 21).

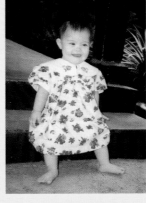

Figure 11.1 Child with Down Syndrome.
(Courtesy of Down Syndrome Association in Singapore)

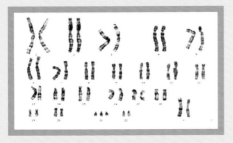

Figure 11.2 Chromosome pattern of a person with Down Syndrome. Arrow points to an extra chromosome number 21.

It is important to know that people with Down Syndrome can also have reasonably long and fulfilling lives.

Throughout the world, the frequency of Down Syndrome is about 1 per 700 births. The risk of having a baby with Down Syndrome increases as the mother's age increases (refer to Fig 11.3).

How Do I Know if My Baby has Down Syndrome?

Until recently, the only factor used to identify women at high risk for Down Syndrome was their age. At age 35, for example, the chance of having a baby with Down Syndrome is about 1 in 250. This has led to many hospitals offering amniocentesis to women over a certain age, usually 35 or 37. There are several other methods available to pick up Down Syndrome. These tests are grouped into **screening** and **diagnostic tests.**

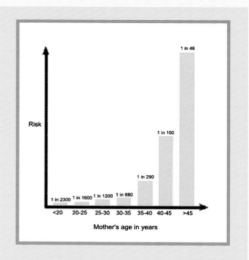

Figure 11.3 Maternal age and the risk of Down Syndrome.

Screening Tests (FTS or MSS)

Screening tests do not tell you if your baby has Down Syndrome. Their purpose is to tell you if your fetus belongs to a *low or high risk group*. If the screening test shows that there is a high risk of your baby being affected, you will be offered a diagnostic test (see below) to confirm it. **Screening tests are non-invasive; hence, there is no risk of miscarriage to the baby**.

- **First trimester screening (FTS)** — This consists of a detailed ultrasound scan of your baby at *11–14 weeks gestation* to measure the nuchal translucency (NT). NT is the skin at the back of your baby's neck (Figure 11.4). If this is increased above the normal range, most babies will still be normal although there is an increased risk of Down Syndrome, heart problem or rare genetic syndrome in some babies. Its accuracy is about 80%, and increases to 90% if maternal blood tests are done as well. This is known as integrated screening.

    A result of 1 in 300 means that 299 out of 300 women with this particular test result will not have an affected baby, and only one will. As you can see, it is not a test for the presence of a Down Syndrome baby, but a way of comparing your chance of having one. So, a 40-year-old woman would be very reassured by a result of 1 in 800 and a 20-year-old woman may opt for amniocentesis if her result was 1 in 100 (Figure 11.5).

- **Maternal serum screening (MSS)** — This measures certain hormones in your blood to determine your risk. These hormones are called alpha-

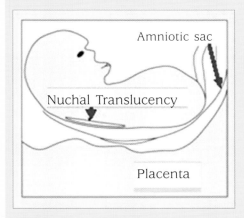 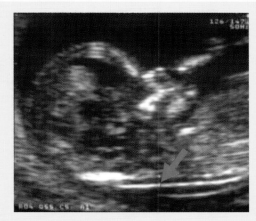

Figure 11.4 Measuring Nuchal Translucency.

fetoprotein, human chorionic gonadotropin, with or without oestriol. Blood is taken at between **15–20 weeks gestation**, and a risk value is calculated, individualized to your age. The result of the test is also expressed in terms of a risk assessment (e.g. 1 in 300).

Overall, about **6–7 out of 10 Down Syndrome babies will be detected by the serum screening**. However, there will still be some that are undetected and will be born to mothers who have had a "low-risk" result.

These screening tests do not guarantee that the baby will be healthy. It only helps to screen for Down Syndrome. If the test result is "low risk", this means that the chance of having this condition is reduced.

Diagnostic Tests (Amniocentesis or Chorionic Villus Sampling)

These are tests that obtain cell samples from the baby and can tell you for sure if the baby is affected with Down Syndrome. It is only performed for high-risk cases detected on screening due to the inherent risks of miscarriage associated with these procedures.

The purpose of diagnosing this condition is to allow the couple the various options of whether to continue with the pregnancy or have an abortion.

IMPORTANT!

It must be clearly understood that the results of screening tests represent risks. Increased risk does not mean that the baby is affected and further diagnostic tests must be done. A low risk does not exclude the possibility of Down Syndrome or other abnormalities as the risk assessment does not detect all affected pregnancies.

- **Amniocentesis** — Down syndrome can be diagnosed early in pregnancy from *15–20 weeks of pregnancy* by amniocentesis. This involves a very fine needle being passed into the womb, under ultrasound guidance, and sampling of the amniotic fluid (water bag) around the baby. It takes about 2–3 weeks for the results to be ready although rapid tests (PCR) can also be done within 3–5 days. Most women do not find it too uncomfortable and takes about 5–10 minutes as an **outpatient procedure**. There is a risk of 0.5% of a spontaneous miscarriage after the procedure, which usually happens within two weeks after the procedure.

- **Chorionic villus sampling (CVS)** — Chorionic villus sampling is another option that is performed even earlier at about *12 weeks of pregnancy*. Like amniocentesis, it is also done under ultrasound guidance. A needle is inserted into the placenta to withdraw the cells through the abdomen or cervix. It allows earlier diagnosis and therefore reduces the anxiety of waiting. The risk of a miscarriage is similar to that of an amniocentesis.

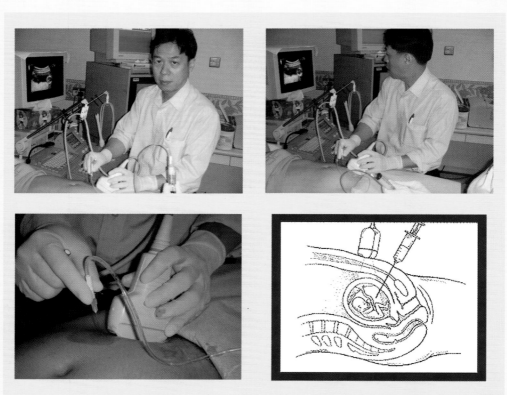

Figure 11.5 Amniocentesis done under ultrasound guidance.

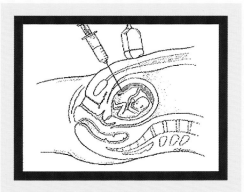

Figure 11.6 Chorionic villus sampling (CVS).

IMPORTANT!

After the amniocentesis or CVS, it is important to return to the hospital immediately if you run a fever, experience any unusual lower abdominal pain, vaginal bleeding or leakage of fluid from the vagina.

- **Fetal blood sampling (FBS)** — This is a test that involves the sampling of fetal blood from the umbilical cord. The risk of miscarriage is much higher at 2–3% and thus, FBS is *rarely performed* for the diagnosis of Down Syndrome.

Table 11.1 Risk of Down Syndrome and genetic problems with mother's age.

Age of mother	Risk of baby with Down Syndrome	Risk of baby with genetic problems
20	1 in 1667	1 in 526
25	1 in 1250	1 in 476
30	1 in 952	1 in 385
35	**1 in 250**	**1 in 192**
37	1 in 224	1 in 127
39	1 in 136	1 in 83
40	1 in 100	1 in 66
42	1 in 63	1 in 42
45	1 in 30	1 in 20

Chapter 12

Thalassemia Tests

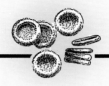

> *At the end of the day, a loving family should find everything forgivable.*
>
> **Mark V. Olsen and Will Sheffer**

Beta thalassemia is an *inherited blood disorder*, which is caused by an abnormal gene. A person with thalassemia is unable to produce normal, functioning hemoglobin in the blood. Hemoglobin carries oxygen from the lungs to all parts of the body. When the body is not able to produce normal, functioning hemoglobin, the affected person suffers from anemia. Thalassemia is passed on from parent to child and can affect both males and females. In Singapore, about 3% of the population are carriers of the thalassemia gene.

NOTE

Alpha thalassemia is a separate condition, which may be tested in specific cases using special DNA test. Alpha thalassemia occurs when one or more of the four alpha blood chain genes fails to function. This condition can be that of a silent carrier (one or two genes deletion), blood-transfusion dependent (three genes deletion) or fatal (four genes deletion).

What are the Types of Thalassemia?

There are two types of thalassemia:

- Thalassemia minor (thalassemia trait)
- Thalassemia major

A person who has inherited one thalassemia gene is said to have thalassemia minor (thalassemia trait). He or she is healthy and leads a normal life.

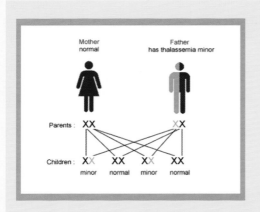

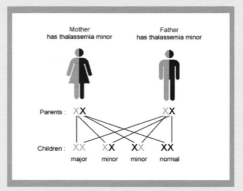

Figure 12.1 Inheritance of thalassemia minor.

Figure 12.2 Inheritance of thalassemia major.

Most people with thalassemia minor do not know they have it. However, the affected persons can pass on the abnormal gene to their children.

Thalassemia major is a severe form of anemia. The affected person has inherited two thalassemia genes, one from each parent. He or she may look normal at birth but within 1–2 years of life, will suffer from severe anemia, which leads to poor growth and development as well as a shorter lifespan.

The affected person will need a blood transfusion every month to sustain life. At present, a bone marrow transplant is the only hope of possible cure for thalassemia major.

How is Thalassemia Inherited?

If only one parent has thalassemia minor, the following can occur:

- 50% chance of having a child with thalassemia minor
- 50% chance of having a normal child
- None of the couple's children will get thalassemia major.

If both parents have thalassemia minor, the following can occur:

- 25% chance of having a child with thalassemia major
- 50% chance of having a child with thalassemia minor
- 25% chance of having a normal child.

The chances are the same with each pregnancy, no matter how many children the couple may have.

Who Should Go for Thalassemia Screening?

Since thalassemia can be passed on from one generation to another, you and your partner should go for a thalassemia screening if you are:

- Planning to get married
- Starting a family.

Thalassemia screening involves a simple blood test which is readily available.

What Should I Do if I Have Thalassemia Minor?

If you or your partner have thalassemia minor, both of you should see a doctor for **genetic counseling** before you plan to get married or have a child. The doctor will explain the risks and discuss the choices you have. He may refer you to the National Thalassemia Registry for further counseling.

The National Thalassemia Registry provides genetic counseling for people with thalassemia and screening for their families.

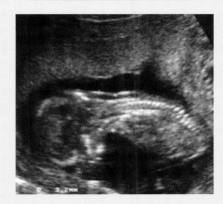

DID YOU KNOW?

- Baby's unique fingerprints start to form at **9 weeks** gestation.
- Baby also starts to urinate after **11 weeks** gestation.
- At **12 weeks** gestation, your baby's crown rump length is 51 mm, about the size of a lime. And your baby will weigh about 18 grams.
- The baby's heartbeat can now be amplified by a Doppler device and you can now hear the baby's heart beat for the first time. It sounds like a galloping horse and is usually between 110–160 beats per minute.

What if I Am Already Pregnant?

If you are already pregnant and both you and your husband have thalassemia, you should go for a prenatal diagnostic test to find out whether your unborn baby has thalassemia major. Prenatal diagnosis can be done by chorionic villus sampling or amniocentesis (see Chapter 11).

Based on the results of the test, the doctor will advise you accordingly.

Chapter 13

Antenatal Blood Tests

> Investigation may be likened to the long months of pregnancy,
> and solving a problem to the day of birth.
> To investigate a problem is, indeed, to solve it.
>
> **Mao Tse-Tung**

These tests are usually done in your pregnancy visits.

Full Blood Count

This measures your hemoglobin levels and enables doctors to detect anemia (low levels of red blood cells that carry oxygen in your body). The most common cause of anemia is **iron deficiency** and you may be prescribed iron supplements.

This test will also enable doctors to screen for **thalassemia**, an inherited genetic condition that may be transmitted to your baby (see Chapter 12). Though less common, your baby may be severely affected if your partner is affected as well. More blood tests such as **hemoglobin electrophoresis** and **DNA tests** may be performed to confirm this diagnosis.

Blood Typing

This tells us several things about your blood. Firstly, it shows which **main blood group** you belong to (A, B, O or AB).

Secondly, it helps to determine your **Rhesus (Rh)** status. You may be Rh positive (majority) or Rh negative (minority). If you happen to be Rh negative, you may require further injections (Rhogam) during the course of your pregnancy to prevent harmful antibodies from being produced that may harm your baby. Your doctor will discuss this in greater detail should you require this.

Hepatitis B Screen

Hepatitis B infection is usually asymptomatic. For the mother, it may affect the liver function and will require long term follow up for any deterioration or cancer change in the liver.

> **NOTE**
>
> If your are a Hepatitis B carrier, a Hepatitis B vaccine and antibodies will be administered to your child immediately after delivery.

This infection can be transmitted to the baby during the birth process. An immunization regime can be started for your baby to reduce this chance of transmission and help prevent your baby from being affected. This minimizes the chance of them developing liver dysfunction and cancer in later years.

Syphilis Screen

Fortunately, this sexually transmitted disease is now rare. However, it is still routinely done as early treatment with antibiotics may prevent stillbirth or deformities.

HIV Screen

The Human Immunodeficiency Virus (HIV) is the virus that causes AIDS (Acquired Immunodeficiency Syndrome). This can affect the immune system and cause eventual death.

If the mother is found to be HIV positive, this can be transmitted to the baby during birth and breastfeeding. Through proper treatment with medications, Cesarean section and avoidance of breastfeeding, the risk of transmission can be reduced to < 1%.

Rubella/German Measles Screen (not routinely done)

Most of the local women would have been vaccinated against this condition when young. If you are immune, you and your baby should be protected even if you come into contact with someone who has a rubella infection during your pregnancy. This is discussed in greater detail in *Chapter 2*.

If the tests indicate that you are not immune, you will be offered a vaccination in the postnatal period.

Oral Glucose Tolerance Test (OGTT)

This tests for diabetes mellitus in pregnancy and will require you to fast overnight. A fasting blood specimen is taken. You will need to drink a glucose solution before measuring your blood glucose levels again two hours later. It is considered *abnormal* if the glucose levels are above a certain level.

Normal OGTT values:
- Fasting glucose level – < 5.5 mmol/L
- 2-hour glucose level – < 7.8 mmol/L

The following group of patients may need OGTT:
- Above 35 years of age
- Persistent glucose in the urine on at least two episodes
- Obesity (weight > 80 kg)
- On long term steroids
- A family history of diabetes in first degree relatives
- A past history of diabetes in pregnancy
- A past history of big babies (> 4 kg)
- Suspected macrosomia (i.e. the baby is considered big for what is expected at the gestational age)
- History of unexplained stillbirth or bad obstetric history

Chapter 14

Antenatal Ultrasound Scans

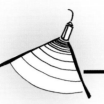

> *Everything about woman is a riddle, and everything about woman has a single solution: that is, pregnancy.*
> **Friedrich Nietzsche**

An ultrasound scan is an assessment tool commonly used by doctors during your pregnancy. It is a **safe and useful** way of obtaining images of your baby and his/her surrounding environment to provide useful information on his/her health (Figure 14.1).

Dating Scan (Week 6–12)

Your first ultrasound scan should be performed in your first trimester of pregnancy. In a usual situation, the scan will show the early pregnancy sac in the

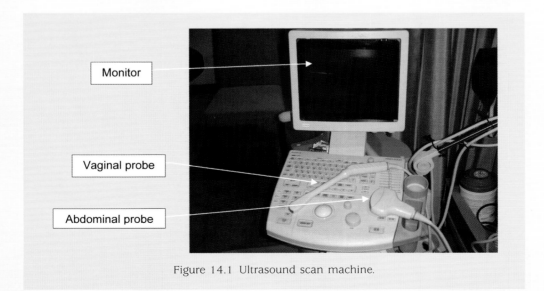

Figure 14.1 Ultrasound scan machine.

womb with the fetus within the sac. This can be seen as early as 5 to 6 weeks of pregnancy. Visualizing the pregnancy in the womb is reassuring, because it confirms that it is in the right location. Although very uncommon, pregnancy can sometimes be implanted in the wrong place like in the fallopian tubes (known as ectopic pregnancy). This happens to 1–2% of all pregnancies. The baby's heartbeat is normally visible by 6 weeks of pregnancy. Sometimes,

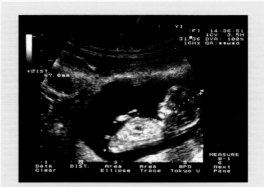

Figure 14.2 Measurement of baby's length (crown rump length) in first trimester.

your doctor may use a vaginal probe for the scan when your pregnancy is about 5 to 6 weeks. **Be assured that vaginal scanning is safe** and will not harm your pregnancy in any way.

The current gestation (age) of your pregnancy can be calculated by taking measurements of your baby during the scan (Figure 14.2 and Table 14.1). Your expected date of delivery (EDD) can then be estimated accurately. This is especially important for your doctor to manage your pregnancy well. It also helps you to plan ahead like informing your employer about maternity leave and making all the necessary arrangements for baby care before the arrival of your baby. Indeed, **the accuracy of the first trimester ultrasound scan is within a week.**

The first trimester ultrasound also allows you to know if you are expecting twins or even triplets.

Table 14.1 Baby's length (crown-rump length) and gestation age.

Crown-Rump Length (cm)	Gestation Age (weeks) = crown-rump length (cm) + 6.5 (rough estimate)
0.8	7
1.0	7.5
1.5	8.0
2.1	9.0
3.1	10.0
4.1	11.0
5.1	12.0

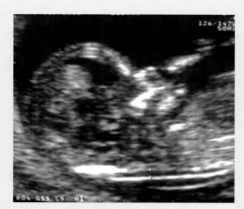

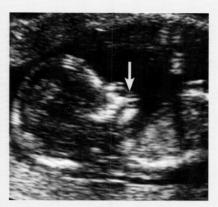

Figure 14.3 Measurement of neck thickness of
baby in Down Syndrome test.

Figure 14.4 Nose bone present.

Nuchal Translucency Scan (Week 11–14)

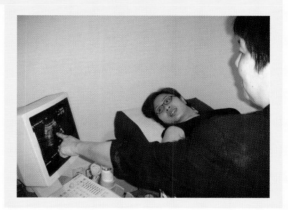

In the recent years, ultrasound scans in the first trimester can be used to assess the risk of your baby being affected by Down Syndrome (Figure 14.3). This is done by a measurement of the skin fold thickness (nuchal translucency) at the back of neck of the baby. If the neck fold is unusually thick, it may indicate that your baby may have Down syndrome (see Chapter 11). Other causes may include heart abnormalities or even other rarer genetic syndromes. This test is quite accurate to detect Down Syndrome as the detection rate is 80% in the hands of experienced doctors. So do consider this test, which is perfectly safe for your baby.

If your baby is in an optimal position, ultrasound examination after 11 weeks may be able to visualize the baby's nose bone (known as nasal bone). The **absence of the nose bone is a worrying sign**, which increases the risk of Down Syndrome.

Screening Scan (Week 18–22)

Being an expectant mother, you will find it reassuring to know that your baby will be born healthy with no congenital deformities. An ultrasound scan can be used for screening to look for abnormalities in the physical structure of

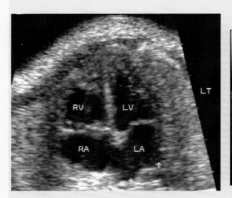

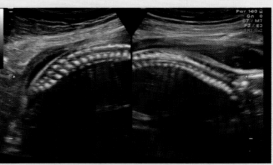

Figure 14.5 Ultrasound scan showing normal heart structures of baby.

Figure 14.6 Ultrasound scan of baby's spine.

the baby, for example in the heart, lungs, spine, brain, long bones in legs or arms, organs in the abdomen like liver, stomach, intestines, kidneys, bladder and even check for cleft lip and palate.

Finding of certain abnormalities during an ultrasound scan may also alert doctors to the possibility of Down Syndrome or other genetic abnormalities in the baby. Further testing can then be done to exclude these. Ultrasound screening for physical abnormalities is usually done during around the fifth month or 20th weeks of your pregnancy.

It is performed by a sonographer or obstetrician, using a fairly advanced ultrasound machine that provides excellent resolution for imaging. The **accuracy of scans is about 70%** in detecting all abnormalities.

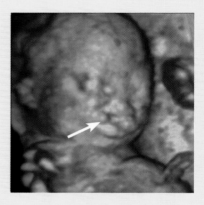

Figure 14.7 3-D ultrasound picture showing a baby's cleft palate.

NOTE

Although a structural screening scan is undertaken, detection of structural problems will never be 100% accurate. Detection rates may vary and be reduced by factors such as maternal obesity, abdominal scars, fetal position and reduced amniotic fluid.

Growth Scan (32–36 weeks)

Later in pregnancy, it is important to monitor your baby's growth. Your doctor

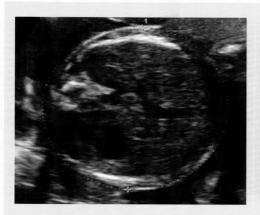

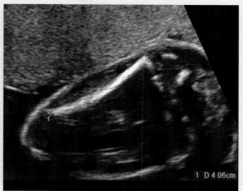

Figure 14.8 Measurement of baby's tummy for growth.

Figure 14.9 Measurement of baby's thigh bone for growth.

will monitor this, most of the time by examining you and measuring the height of your tummy during your regular visits.

Ultrasound scan from late second trimester may help to confirm that your baby is growing well (Figure 14.8). We can also tell if the amniotic fluid in the "water-bag" is sufficient for the baby. This tells us about the health status of baby.

This scan is also useful to determine your baby's position and the placenta location in the womb. This will help your doctor decide if it would be safe to deliver your baby through the normal birth passage, or if a Cesarean section may be necessary.

Doppler Scan

Sometimes, a more specialized mode of ultrasound called a Doppler ultrasound scan may be used for more specific conditions (Figure 14.10). For example, when the growth of the baby is reduced or anemia (low hemoglobin) is suspected in the baby. Doppler scan can help to provide additional information on the blood flow status of the placenta and the health status of the baby.

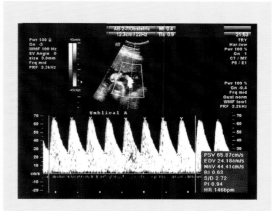

Figure 14.10 Umbilical artery doppler study.

DID YOU KNOW?

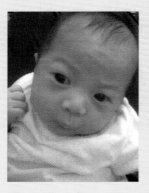

- You may be able to determine your baby's sex with a ultrasound scan after 16–20 weeks gestation.
- All your baby's organs are formed by 16 weeks gestation.
- At 16 weeks gestation, your baby weighs 146 g and is about 12 cm long, about the size of an avocado.
- Your baby can now hear your voice and heartbeat. Music and mother's voice are calming to the baby.
- Your baby can also make sucking, swallowing and breathing movements.
- Your baby's heart is now pumping about 6 gallons of blood a day!

FREQUENTLY ASKED QUESTIONS

1. **What do I expect at an ultrasound scan?**

   You will be asked to lie on a couch, back down. The lights will be dimmed so that it is easier for the doctor to see the images of your baby. An ultrasound scan is done with placing the scan probe on your tummy. Before that some gel will be applied on your tummy. In the early weeks of pregnancy, a probe placed through the vagina may be used to see your baby clearly.

2. **When should I go for my first ultrasound scan in pregnancy?**

   Having a scan during the first trimester (first 12 weeks) is very useful for you to know your gestation and due date. This is important for your doctor for optimal management of your pregnancy.

   However, having a scan too early in pregnancy will not yield the necessary information, as the developing baby is not seen on scan until 5–6 weeks of pregnancy (from the first day of your last menses if you have a regular 28-day cycles). Measurements of the baby can be done more accurately after 8 weeks gestation. The most ideal time for dating scan is between 8 to 12 weeks of pregnancy.

3. Is an ultrasound scan safe for my baby?

While the safety of ultrasound scans in pregnancy is endorsed by professional experts and is now a common tool in pregnancy assessment, it is still important to exercise prudency. You should understand the purpose and reason for each ultrasound scan. Also, doctors would ensure that each ultrasound examination is done carefully within a reasonable time.

4. What is a 3D scan and do I need one?

A 3D ultrasound can furnish us with a three-dimensional image of the fetus. The transducer takes a series of images and the computer processes these images and presents them as a three-dimensional image. These costly scans are regarded as "social scans" at the present moment and generally do not add value to the diagnosis of fetal structural problems. Occasionally, it can help to delineate small structural problems such as abnormality in the fingers or toes and minor skin defects. Most hospitals do not offer 3D scans as a routine scan.

5. What is the chance of my baby having a major fetal abnormality?

The risk in the general population that a fetus has a **major structural birth defect is 2–3%**. While not all abnormalities can be identified by ultrasound scans, many can be. When a comprehensive examination of the fetus is normal, the risk of a major abnormality is about 1%. Some structural problems like heart defects may recur in subsequent pregnanices. Do consult your doctor who will counsel you on the risks accordingly.

Chapter 15

Do's and Don'ts in Pregnancy

 Love the moment. Flowers grow out of dark moments.
Therefore, each moment is vital. It affects the whole.
Life is a succession of such moments and to live each,
is to succeed.

Corita Kent

Food, Smoking, Alcohol and Recreational Drugs in Pregnancy

Dos:

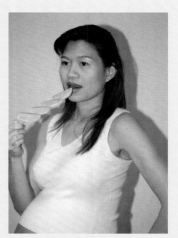

- **Folic acid supplementation**
  Folic acid is a type of vitamin B that is needed for the formation of blood cells and the development of baby's nervous system. It has been shown to **reduce the chance of a baby having brain and spinal cord defects**. A simple way is to take a 5 mg folate supplement for the first 12 weeks of pregnancy.
- Eat a variety of healthy food rich in iron, calcium and folate. (See Chapter 25 on Nutrition during pregnancy — eating right for two.)

Don'ts:

- **Smoking**
  Smoking is associated with adverse effects on both the pregnant mother and her fetus. It can cause an **increased risk of miscarriage, prema-**

ture separation of placenta, premature birth and a low birth-weight baby*. There is also a long-term relationship with *decreased intellectual development* of the infant and *increased risk of Sudden Infant Death Syndrome* (cot death).

Much less is known about the consequences of exposure to passive smoke during fetal development. However, the performance of children of passive smokers was found, in most areas, to be between that of active smoking and nonsmoking mothers.

- **Alcohol consumption**
  Alcohol consumption in pregnancy is linked to infants showing *behavioral and learning difficulties*. Excessive alcohol consumption is associated with *Fetal Alcohol Syndrome* (FAS) where the infant may have varying negative effects including congenital malformations and mental retardation.

- **Caffeine**
  Safety of caffeine consumption during pregnancy is *controversial*. Some studies suggest that a modest caffeine intake of two cups of coffee per day presents a slight risk to the fetus, but others do not. There is some evidence that consuming larger amounts of caffeine daily during pregnancy may increase risks of *miscarriage, preterm delivery and low birth weight*, but these studies are non-conclusive.

  We recommend limiting any drinks containing caffeine such as coffee, tea and cola to a *maximum of two cups per day* for the safety of your baby.

- **Diet**
  Do not focus on a weight loss regime during pregnancy.

- **Recreational drugs**
  If you have been abusing recreational or "lifestyle" drugs like cocaine, heroine, amphetamine ("Ecstasy pill"), or marijuana, it is the most appropriate time for you to quit totally once you are pregnant. Continuing to consume these substances is harmful to your developing baby. *They are known to cause miscarriage, bleeding in the placenta, stillbirth, low birth-weight baby and even mental retardation of baby*. Birth defects associated with maternal cocaine use include abnormalities of the brain, skull, face, eyes, heart, limbs, intestines, genitals and urinary tract.

  Discuss this with your doctor so that appropriate help and support can be rendered to you.

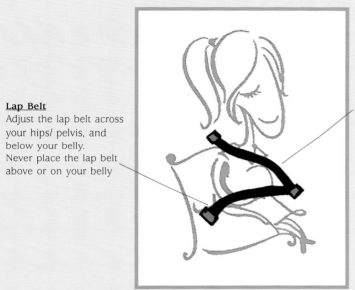

Shoulder Belt
Place the shoulder belt across your chest, between your breasts, and away from your neck. Never place the shoulder belt behind your back or under your arm.

Lap Belt
Adjust the lap belt across your hips/ pelvis, and below your belly.
Never place the lap belt above or on your belly

Figure 15.1 The right way to wear a seat belt during pregnancy.

Travel in Pregnancy

- Flying is not contraindicated in an uncomplicated pregnancy. You must be well with no abdominal pain or bleeding. Domestic travel is usually permitted until 36 weeks gestation whereas international travel may be curtailed after 32 weeks of pregnancy. This is due to the risk of preterm delivery.
- Traveling should be done mostly in the second trimester when the pregnant woman is more comfortable and the risk of miscarriage and preterm delivery are lower.
- It is important to take deep vein thrombosis (blood clots in the legs) precautions such as getting a seat with more leg room, interval walking in the aisles or toilet breaks, leg massages or wearing thrombosis deterrent stockings. Prevent dehydration by taking enough fluids orally and avoiding alcohol.
- You can **consider meningococcal and rabies vaccines** if these diseases are endemic in the country you are traveling to. The **safety of vaccines for yellow fever, Hepatitis A and typhoid is not yet established in pregnancy**.
- When traveling in a car, always wear a seat belt to protect you and your unborn baby. The seat belt should be a 3-point restraint with a lap and shoulder belts.

- Wear your seat belt correctly. The lap belt should go under your belly, across your hips and as high as possible on your thighs. The shoulder strap should go between your breasts and off to the side of your belly. Seat belt straps should fit snugly and never go directly across your tummy. (Figure 15.1)

Carrying Heavy Objects in Pregnancy

- It is common to hear that it is unsafe to lift heavy things in pregnancy. However, the risk of injury is usually directed at the mother and not the baby. The increase in the level of hormones during pregnancy causes the ligaments to soften, which leads to joints that may be less stable.
- Also, the center of gravity of the pregnant mother has shifted which puts more stress on her back. These two factors make the mother more susceptible to injury when lifting heavy things.

Clothing in Pregnancy

- The womb does not grow out of the pelvis until 12 weeks of pregnancy and most women will still get away with wearing their normal clothes until then.
- By 14–16 weeks, the belly starts protruding and you will need to wear looser or more elasticized pants or skirts. Between 18–22 weeks, the waistline thickens, and the clothes need to accommodate this to maintain comfort.
- Temperature increases during pregnancy and thus light, breathable clothing made of wool or cotton is preferred. Shorts/skirts or pants with elastic or drawstring waist made from stretchy materials that can grow with your waist is preferable.
- As long as pregnant women are comfortable in their clothing and the clothing is not too restrictive or tight, it should not impede the development of the baby.
- Exposing the belly has no known adverse effects on the developing baby.
- Normal underwear can be worn during pregnancy. However, some women prefer oversized underwear to pull up over their bump. During pregnancy, body temperature increases and vaginal discharge changes. Pregnant women are thus more prone to fungal and bacterial infections. Cotton underwear will keep the perineal area ventilated and discourage growth of these organisms.
- Avoid wearing tight socks or half leg stockings during pregnancy as these can reduce blood circulation from the feet and lower legs, thus increasing swelling, fluid retention and aggravating varicose veins.

Footwear in Pregnancy

- Your feet increase in size during pregnancy due to water retention in the legs. Also, pregnant women are prone to falling and tripping due to changes in centre of gravity and dynamics.
- Flat and low-heeled shoes are preferable. Backless shoes made of flexible material can accommodate to changes your feet.

Hair-Dyeing, Hair Rebonding and Perming in Pregnancy

- The concern about exposures to hair dye and hair straightening agents is that there may be absorption of chemicals into the bloodstream at the time of use. However, most chemicals are cleared from the bloodstream fairly quickly. Unfortunately, there have been only very few studies on the use of such products during pregnancy to quantify the risk of hair dye to a developing baby.
- While no one can provide data about timing and safety, **avoid dyeing or rebonding the hair** once the woman has conceived.
- **Perming hair during the second and third trimesters of pregnancy is a safe procedure** and can make caring for hair less time consuming and easier. There are no studies that indicate perming of hair during pregnancy is detrimental to the fetus.

Keeping Pets in Pregnancy

- **Pregnancy and your dog**
  Dogs are usually safe for you and your developing baby. However, be careful of large dogs, which may jump on your tummy while you are lying down or sitting.

- **Pregnancy and your cat**
  Cats may transmit toxoplasmosis (a parasitic infection). Toxoplasmosis can cause premature delivery, serious malformations of baby and low birth-weight.

  Transmission usually occurs from contact with feline feces. Outdoor cats are more likely to have toxoplasmosis than cats that remain strictly indoors. Since cats may use both litter boxes and outdoor sand and soil, you can become infected after changing a contaminated litter box, digging or gardening outside, or eating unwashed contaminated fruits and vegetables.

  If you are immune to toxoplasmosis by previous infection before pregnancy, then you are not likely to be infected again. Thus, if you are a cat owner and trying to get pregnant, ask your doctor for a simple blood test (antibodies level) to check if you are immune to toxoplasmosis. Unfortunately, there is no useful vaccine against toxoplasmosis.

Eat only well-cooked meat. Avoid dried raw meats such as beef jerky. Wash the fruits and vegetables before eating them and all utensils after preparing raw meat, seafood, fruits and vegetables.

- **Pregnancy and your pet bird**
  Birds can transmit infections like **campylobacter and salmonella. They can cause miscarriage in early pregnancy or stillbirth in advanced pregnancy.**

  It is useful to bring your pet bird to your veterinarian to check for such infections. Inform your doctor that you have a pet bird in the house.

  Always wash your hands thoroughly with soap and hot water following any handling of the bird or its cage. Avoid changing the birdcage if possible.

- **Pregnancy and farm animals**
  Farm animals are known to transmit listeria, campylobacter and also salmonella infections. Listeria infection can cause severe infection, miscarriage or stillbirth.

  Thus, try to **avoid leisure farm visits**. Always wash your hands thoroughly with soap and hot water following any contact with farm animals or their living areas. Do not feed the animals or handle the dead animals. Drink only pasteurized milk as this would eliminate the risk of food-borne listeriosis.

Prenatal Stimulation

Prenatal stimulation uses various stimuli such as classical music and the mother's voice. The baby learns to recognize and respond to different stimuli, which may encourage physical, mental, and sensory development. Babies may benefit from stimulation *as early as the third month of pregnancy*. Once babies develop hearing in the fifth month, music is excellent for aural stimulation and to soothe the baby.

- **Does it really work?**
  Some studies have revealed that stimulated babies exhibit enhanced hearing, linguistic, and motor development. In general, they sleep better, are more alert, confident and content than infants who were not stimulated. They also show superior learning capacity and calm down

more easily when they hear familiar sounds they heard while in the womb.

Stimulated babies and their families showed more intense bonding and greater family cohesion. Prenatal stimulation provides a lasting foundation for loving communication and healthy parent-child relationships.

- **Is over-stimulation a concern?**
  Over-stimulation may cause confusion. When babies become overwhelmed by too much stimulation, they may stop responding. Stick to **moderate** levels of stimulation if you desire.

Use of Computers in Pregnancy

All electrical equipment can produce low frequency (non-ionizing) radiation. Computer monitors have internal shielding that reduces non-ionizing radiation to safe levels. Computer users who sit at typical distances from their monitors receive extremely low exposures. Current research suggests there are few, if any, health effects caused by non-ionizing radiation among computer users.

Many pregnant mothers are worried that the low-level electromagnetic fields (non-ionizing radiation) produced by computer monitors could cause miscarriage or harm an unborn baby. It is heartening to know that studies have shown no evidence that this is the case.

However, avoid sitting in front of a computer for hours at a time because you may experience *worsening of your backache*. If you must spend extended periods in front of the computer, take frequent short breaks to walk, stretch and move to prevent blood clots in the legs (deep vein thrombosis).

X-Rays in Pregnancy

- X-rays or Computed Tomography scans are to be **avoided** in pregnancy unless the benefits outweigh the risks of radiation to the fetus which can cause developmental malformations and childhood cancers.
- The amount of radiation used during a CT scan is considered minimal and therefore, the risk for radiation exposure is low.
- Inadvertent exposure to X-ray in pregnancy, even in the first trimetser, may **not** necessarily be an indication to terminate the pregnancy.
- **Avoid X-rays** during pregnancy unless ordered by your doctor. You will usually be given **a lead apron** to shield the developing fetus if an X-ray is a must during pregnancy.

FREQUENTLY ASKED QUESTIONS

1. Can I go for massage and aromatherapy during pregnancy?

Massage is a wonderful way to unwind tired muscles and pamper you. The massage table should have a cutout for your belly. Otherwise, you can position yourself with pillows so you are slightly on your side, or use a massage chair. However, ***massage of the tummy or breasts can cause contractions of the womb***. If you notice strong contractions, stop that part of the massage.

You may find that you are more sensitive to smells than usual. Aromatherapy is fine as long as it is pleasant for you. However, essential oils are absorbed through your skin into the bloodstream. Until more is known, *avoid extensive skin contact with essential oils*, especially in the first trimester while the baby's organs are developing.

2. Can I enter a sauna or steam room during pregnancy?

High fever in early pregnancy is bad for the developing baby as it increases the chances of miscarriage and birth defects like spinal cord and brain malformation. Thus, *all treatments that raise your body temperature should be off limits during pregnancy*. These include the sauna, steam room and hot tub. Warm baths are fine as long as they are not super hot, since water cools off fairly quickly.

3. Can I begin a weight loss regime in pregnancy? Would being underweight cause a problem in pregnancy?

Women who are severely underweight (body mass index < 19 kg/m^2) during pregnancy and who are not eating enough are more likely to have a **baby who is small and of low birth-weight**. This can have serious long-term effects on the baby's health. Most pregnant women should expect a weight gain of **10–12 kg** throughout the entire pregnancy.

Take a balanced diet during pregnancy consisting of calories, carbohydrates, proteins and fibers. **Dieting is a no-no in pregnancy**. Your baby needs you to eat! Your baby depends on you for its nourishment. Remember that if you eat well, your baby eats well and if you starve, your baby starves.

4. With symptoms of pregnancy like shortness of breath and constant urination, are there any ways to get good night sleep?

Pregnancy is demanding both physically and emotionally. The increasing size of your belly makes it hard to find a comfortable sleeping position.

If you have always been a back or stomach sleeper, it may be difficult to get used to sleeping on your side as recommended by your doctor. Also, as the growing womb presses on your bladder, you experience more trips to the bathroom, day and night. See your doctor to exclude urinary tract infection if you experience a burning sensation when urinating.

Try to get into the habit of sleeping on your side early in your pregnancy. Lying on your side with your knees bent is likely to be the most comfortable position as your pregnancy progresses. It also makes your heart's job easier because it prevents the baby's weight from applying pressure to the large vein (the inferior vena cava). Alternatively, use a pillow to keep yourself propped up on one side. Some doctors specifically **recommend that pregnant women sleep on the left side**. This is because your liver is on the right side and lying on your left side helps keep the womb off your liver. Ask what your doctor recommends — but in most cases, lying on either side should be fine.

Cut out caffeinated drinks like coke, coffee and tea from your diet as much as possible especially at night. Avoid drinking a lot of fluids or eating a full meal within a few hours of going to bed at night. This might give you a better sleep with less interruptions to wake up at night to go to the bathroom.

5. **Are electronic massage chairs and foot reflexology safe during pregnancy?**

Unfortunately, there is **insufficient data and research** done at this moment to address the safety of massage chairs and foot reflexology during pregnancy.

6. **Can I have facial treatments during pregnancy?**

The surge of hormones in pregnancy may worsen acne on your face. Thus, facial treatments to treat acne may not be effective. Do pamper yourself with a facial treatment if you find it relaxing and reduce your stress during pregnancy.

Avoid using facial products that contain relaxation oils as they may precipitate womb contractions.

7. **Can I have LASIK surgery to correct my eyesight during pregnancy?**

It is advisable not to have LASIK surgery during pregnancy. During pregnancy, your refraction may be different due to hormonal changes. Also there is the rare possibility that your response to the surgery might not be usual. There is no harm of the surgery to the fetus but your results may be affected. LASIK surgery can be done at least **six weeks** after breastfeeding.

8. **Does pregnancy affect my eyesight?**
Some women may experience worsening of myopia during pregnancy but they would return to the same level of myopia after delivery. Pushing during normal natural birth has not been shown to cause worsening of myopia and retinal detachment.

Visual changes in pregnancy are common, and many are specifically associated with the pregnancy itself. Serious retinal detachments and blindness occur more frequently during pre-eclampsia (high blood pressure). A decreased tolerance to contact lenses is also common during pregnancy; therefore, it is advisable to wear contact lenses only after delivery.

9. **How does fear or loud noises affect my pregnancy? Will watching horror movies affect my baby?**
Fear activates your nervous system to produce adrenaline hormones. Adrenaline will increase your heart rate and your breathing becomes more shallow and faster. Your blood pressure will increase as well.

Watching horror movies in pregnancy is more of a cultural taboo. There is no scientific proof to show its harmful effects on the baby. But fear would evoke the adrenaline gush as described. Loud noises do not usually affect your fetus as he/she is surrounded by amniotic fluid and buffered from the noises.

As we encourage all pregnant women to be calm and relaxed and think of happy things, listening to calm music and watching nice entertainment programs will be a better alternative.

10. **Is acupuncture safe for pregnancy?**
Advocates of acupuncture treatment suggest that acupuncture during pregnancy is beneficial for both mother and baby. During the first trimester, acupuncture may reduce morning sickness and fatigue. During the second trimester, acupuncture can help maintain balance. In the **third trimester**, acupuncture can provide relief from backache and joint pain. Acupuncture is also used during labor for pain relief.

However, if you are considering acupuncture during pregnancy, you should discuss it with your obstetrician.

11. **Does pregnancy affect my sleeping pattern?**

Many women report daytime sleepiness during pregnancy. Try to fit in a quick nap at lunchtime if possible. Most over-the-counter and prescription sleep medications are off-limits when you are pregnant, especially during the first trimester as they may cause fetal malformations and mental retardation. Try activities such as yoga, deep breathing, a relaxing massage or taking a warm bath before bedtime, to get a better night's sleep.

12. **Is it safe for me to paint my baby's room during pregnancy?**

Paint toxicity depends on the chemicals and solvents found in the paint along with the amount of exposure. There are currently no studies that look into the effects of household painting on pregnancy and the developing baby. Household painting involves very low levels of exposure to toxic chemicals. However, we still recommend you to avoid painting if possible.

Also, lead based paint was often used prior to the 1970s, so you should avoid getting involved with removing old paint in an older house because of the risk of lead exposure.

13. **Is it safe to use mobile phones during pregnancy?**

Many mothers are concerned about the possible harmful effects of cell-phone radiation. Unfortunately, there is **insufficient scientific research** done to comment on the safety of cellphone usage at the moment.

14. **I reached an airport X-ray screener that is used to screen our carry-on items. What is the radiation exposure?**

Airport X-ray machines to screen briefcases and packages give much lower doses of radiation than X-ray machines in hospitals and medical clinics — **almost immeasurable**. They are designed this way because they do not have to see in such detail.

15. **Does passing through the airport security pose a risk to my baby during pregnancy?**

Passing through an airport security portal has not been shown to pose a risk to a pregnant woman or her unborn child. The metal detector is not known to pose any health risk to individuals. The devices used to scan your carry-ons are very well shielded so there is no risk passing through the airport security.

Chapter 16

Exercise in Pregnancy

> Physical fitness is not only one of the most important keys to a healthy body, it is the basis of dynamic and creative intellectual activity.
>
> **John F. Kennedy**

We recommend that you maintain an active lifestyle and continue to exercise in **moderation** throughout your entire pregnancy, unless otherwise instructed by your doctor.

Exercise prepares you for the physical demands of labor and motherhood. It also helps to improve your posture and reduces backache, constipation and leg swelling. You will feel less tired and sleep better. You will also gain less body fat. If you are a diabetic in pregnancy, you will be able to control your blood sugar better with exercise.

You will also find that you return to your pre-pregnancy fitness and healthy weight faster after your delivery!

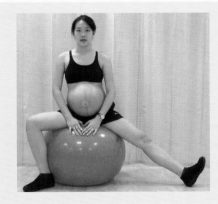

Figure 16.1 Low impact aerobics

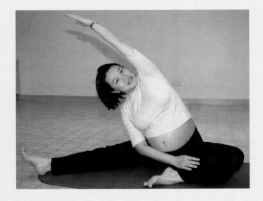

Figure 16.2 Simple stretching

Body changes in pregnancy that affect your ability to exercise

Body changes	Risk during exercise in pregnancy
Shift in center of gravity due to the growing belly	Stress on lower back and pelvis. Risk of losing balance and falling.
Joint laxity caused by hormonal changes during pregnancy	Risk of joint injuries, e.g. sprains.
Weight gain	Greater strain on joints and muscles.
Increase in basal metabolic rate and core body temperature	Risk of overheating (hyperthermia). Body temperature in excess of $39.2\,°C$ may cause malformations in baby in the first trimester. **Avoid overheating.**
The growing fetus receives its oxygen and nutrients supply via the placenta	Exercise increases blood flow to the working muscles and away from other parts of the body. Blood flow to the placenta may be compromised at high intensity exercise and during dehydration.

Plan Your Exercise Routine

- **Get medical clearance**

  If you have any obstetric or medical conditions such as persistent vaginal bleeding, twin pregnancies, history of premature labor, high blood pressure or heart disease, check with your obstetrician before beginning an exercise program. If you have no serious medical problems and have an uncomplicated pregnancy, it is safe for you to perform some form of exercise in moderation.

- **Type of exercises**

  Most forms of exercises are safe during pregnancy. **Walking** is a great exercise for beginners. It is a good form of aerobic exercise with minimal stress on your joints. Other suitable exercise for pregnant women include **swimming, cycling on a stationary bike, yoga, stretching, low-impact aerobics and pilates.** If you were a runner before pregnancy, you should be able to keep running during pregnancy but you may need to reduce your mileage, speed, intensity and go for easier routes.

  Avoid contact sports, competitive sports, activities that involve jumping, jarring motions or demand rapid changes of direction. After the first three months of pregnancy, it is best to avoid performing activities while lying on your back, as the weight of the womb may interfere with blood circulation. Also, avoid standing still for long periods of time. Strength training is safe during pregnancy and helps to keep your muscles strong and prevent aches and pains which are common in pregnancy.

- **Exercise schedule**
  You should aim for 30 minutes of exercise at most, if not all, days of the week. Start slowly if it has been some time since you last worked out. Begin with five minutes of exercise a day and add five minutes each week until you can stay active for 30 minutes a day. If you have been exercising before pregnancy, it is probably safe for you to work out at the same level while you are pregnant — as long as you feel comfortable and your obstetrician has given you the green light.

- **Exercise intensity**
  Avoid exercising to the point of exhaustion. Maintain a moderate intensity — if you are able to talk normally while exercising, your exercise intensity is at an acceptable level. Do not try to exercise beyond your current fitness level. Rest frequently if you are feeling breathless. Work at a level of intensity below your threshold.

- **Warm up and cool down**
  To prepare your muscles and joints, begin each exercise session with a 5 to 10 minute warm up. This consists of light activities such as slow walking and stretching exercises. After exercising, cool down by slowly reducing your activity and performing stretching exercises to reduce muscle soreness.

Additional Points To Note Before You Exercise

- **Hydration**
  Drink plenty of water before, during and after exercise to prevent dehydration and overheating. Avoid exercising under the hot sun and reduce your exercise intensity on hot days.

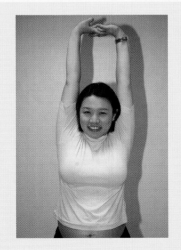

Figure 16.3 Cooling down after exercise.

- **Nutrition**
  Make sure you consume adequate calories to support your baby's growth and development and your daily needs.

- **Clothing**
  Wear comfortable and light clothing that will help you to remain cool. Wear a bra that fits well and gives lots of support to protect your breasts.

Listen to Your Body

Do not force yourself to exercise if you do not feel like it or are too tired on a particular day. Expect a decline in overall activity and fitness level as your pregnancy progresses. This is normal as the physical demands of pregnancy increases. Pay attention to your body while exercising. Be aware of the warning signs (see below), stop exercising and see your obstetrician if you notice any of these symptoms.

Warning Signs:

- Vaginal bleeding
- Decreased fetal movements
- Fluid leaking from the vagina
- Painful womb contractions
- Chest pain
- Dizziness or feeling faint
- Shortness of breath
- Headache
- Calf pain or swelling
- Excessive fatigue

After the Baby is Born

Regular exercise after childbirth benefits new mothers as it promotes the post-partum recovery process, and the return to pre-pregnancy weight and fitness level. It also increases your energy to cope with the demands of motherhood and reduces stress and depression.

If your pregnancy and delivery was uncomplicated, you may begin a light exercise program after six weeks. However, if your delivery was complicated or if you had a cesarean delivery, consult your obstetrician before resuming physical activity. Gradually return to more vigorous activities or your pre-pregnancy exercise levels when you feel stronger. ***Try to exercise after breastfeeding when your breasts are less full and heavy***.

Abdominal Exercise after Delivery

Abdominal exercise can be performed safely after delivery to reduce back pain. Abdominal muscles are usually split in the middle by the growing belly. If you had a Cesarean section, they will be split during the surgery as well. It is important that they are healed before you progress to more demanding abdominal exercises such as sit ups and crunches. Meanwhile you can try this simple exercise to tone your tummy after delivery.

- Breathe out and draw your belly button back towards your spine.
- Hold this position and breathe lightly. Count to 10.
- Relax and repeat up to 10 times (one set).
- Do as many sets per day as possible.
- You can perform this exercise sitting, standing or on your hands and knees.

DID YOU KNOW?

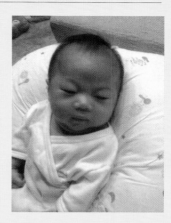

- Small baby kicks may be felt by the mother after **18 weeks** gestation.
- At **20 weeks** gestation, baby weighs about 300 grams and is about 16 cm long.
- Baby also starts to develop sleep wake patterns similar to that of a newborn.
- A layer of white creamy vernix coats your baby's body, protecting your baby's skin from the long months of submersion in amniotic fluid.

Chapter 17
Aqua Exercise in Pregnancy

> *It is exercise alone that supports the spirits, and keeps the mind in vigor.*
>
> **Marcus Tullius Cicero**

E xercise during pregnancy prepares your body physically to undergo vast adaptations during your childbearing period, from conception to postpartum. It also speeds up the restoration of your physical condition.

Exercise in Water

Aqua exercise is a low impact workout that helps to maintain flexibility, enhance stamina and strengthen muscles, joints and bones with minimal risk of injury.

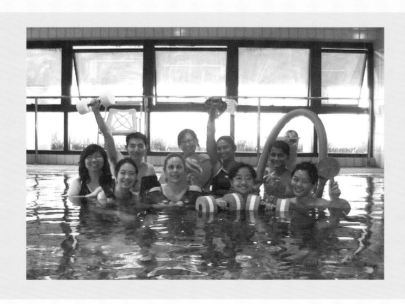

Water exercise in pregnancy does not require the pregnant woman to know how to swim.

Effects of Exercising In Water

The buoyancy in water places less stress on joints and ligaments as compared to exercising on land. This will also reduce the risk of joint injury. Your weight is well supported in water and thus, there is less discomfort during the exercise.

In aqua exercise, there is also less muscle soreness after exercising when compared to exercising on land. Exercising in water is also a good way to train your balance as the abdominals and back muscles stabilize you while you are in the water.

The hydrostatic pressure of water also decreases edema or swelling of the legs. In addition, exercising in water against its natural resistance causes you to expand a great amount of energy.

Additional Benefits of Aqua Exercise During Pregnancy

The buoyancy in water provides relief from the extra weight that the pregnant woman is carrying. It will also reduce lower backache related to the pregnancy. The edema (swelling) of the legs will also be reduced. Exercise in a warm pool will reduce muscle spasms. Aqua exercise expands a greater amount of energy, which is ideal for weight control. It has been shown that exercise in water may increase the blood flow to the womb and thus, to the baby.

Who is *Not* Suitable for Aqua Exercise in Pregnancy?

If you have an acute fear or phobia of water, vaginal infection or itchy skin conditions, aqua exercise is ***not*** suitable for you. Do consult your doctor if this form of exercise is suitable for you.

Chapter 18

Pelvic Floor Exercises

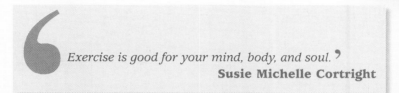

> *Exercise is good for your mind, body, and soul.*
> **Susie Michelle Cortright**

What are Pelvic Floor Muscles?

The pelvic floor muscles form the support of the organs in the pelvis like intestines, urinary bladder ("urine bag"), urethra ("urine tube") and uterus (womb). They also assist the tight closure of the sphincters of the urethra and anus, so that there will be no leakage of urine or feces (Figure 18.1).

In the absence or weakening of these supports, there would be prolapse (sagging) of the womb, bladder and rectum. There may also be incontinence (leakage) of urine when laughing, sneezing or even during brisk walking or exercise.

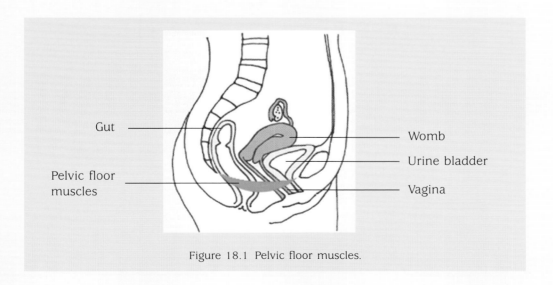

Figure 18.1 Pelvic floor muscles.

Pregnancy and its Effect on the Pelvic Floor Muscles

The pelvic floor muscle stretches during pregnancy as a result of hormonal changes and increase weight in the womb. Furthermore, these muscles stretch further during vaginal delivery as the baby passes through the natural birth passage.

All these forces result in weakening of the pelvic floor muscles which compromises its support and sphincter function. This may lead to symptoms of urinary incontinence (leakage) or prolapse of the pelvic organs as described above (see Chapter 52).

Pelvic Floor Exercises (PFE)

Pelvic floor exercises (PFE) are a set of exercises which aim to strengthen the pelvic floor muscles. PFE has been shown to reduce the incidence of prolapse and urinary leakage, especially after the delivery of your baby.

When to Start PFE in Pregnancy?

You should initiate these exercises from the start of your pregnancy and they must be continued **daily** throughout the entire pregnancy.

How to Perform Pelvic Floor Exercises?

> ### IMPORTANT!
>
> **Do not** breathe in or squeeze your abdominals. **Do not** hold your breath. **Do not** squeeze your thigh or buttock muscles.

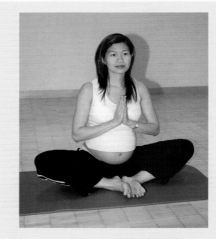

Figure 18.2: Pelvic floor exercise.

> ### IMPORTANT!
>
> A valsalva maneuver could be wrongly performed instead of pelvic floor muscle tightening. This will further stretch and weaken the muscle. Please check with your doctor or physiotherapist for the correct technique.

Imagine that your urinary bladder feels full and you are unable to locate the toilet. Gently squeeze your pelvic floor muscles together right from the anus to the urethra to prevent the urine from leaking. You should feel the whole pelvic floor tightening up.

Exercise 1:	Exercise 2:
• Hold contraction.	• Fast contraction.
• Squeeze the muscle and hold for 10 seconds.	• Squeeze and relax the muscles quickly.
• Relax and rest up to 10 seconds.	• Repeat 10 times.
• Repeat 10 times.	

Do both exercises together each time. Repeat these exercises regularly throughout the day. It can be done in any position — lying, sitting, standing or even walking.

NEVER practice while passing urine. Stopping the stream of urine intermittently may result in incomplete voiding.

Pelvic Floor Exercises After Delivery

When continued into the postnatal period after your delivery, PFE help to reduce perineal swelling by improving circulation through the muscle pump action. They also reduce pain in the perineal area by preventing muscle spasm and tension.

PFE strengthens the weakened muscles to regain its original support and sphincter function as soon as possible. The weakened muscles would not "build" back its strength on its own if these exercises are not done.

The Ultimate Pelvic Floor Test

This test can be performed after six weeks post delivery. On a full bladder, jump up and down for ten times. Also, cough strongly for ten times.

If there is *no* urine leakage, your pelvic floor muscles are considered strong!

DID YOU KNOW?

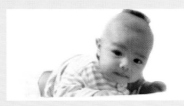

- At **24 weeks gestation**, baby weighs an average of 500 grams and is about 30 cm long.
- Your baby's lungs start branching into air sacs and producing **surfactant**, a substance that prevents the lungs from collapsing during exhalation and allows your baby to breathe properly when born.

Chapter 19

Sex in Pregnancy

> *You must begin to think of yourself as becoming the person you want to be.*
>
> **David Viscott**

B eing pregnant does not diminish the desire for intimacy between couples. However many couples have concerns that sexual intercourse may harm the pregnancy in some way.

Is Sex Safe in Pregnancy?

Yes, if you are having an uneventful pregnancy. Sex is safe and has no harmful effects on the pregnancy or the fetus. Although there are concerns that the womb may experience contractions after an orgasm, these are harmless in most instances and would not precipitate labor in a pregnant woman.

Will it Hurt My Baby?

No, sex in an uncomplicated pregnancy is safe and will not hurt your baby. The baby is surrounded by an "amniotic sac" as well as a thick womb wall which cushions it from any motion. The mucus plug in the cervix prevents any infection from entering the uterus.

Will My Sex Drive Be Affected in Pregnancy?

This varies among different women. As a general rule, the sex drive increases in most women in the second trimester as they are able to adapt better physically and emotionally to their pregnancy by then. Some women feel more attractive during pregnancy, and want to be more intimate with their partners. Conversely, some couples may be concerned about the possibility of sex endangering the pregnancy. This results in decreased libido.

Normal pregnancy conditions like nausea, vomiting and tiredness in the first trimester may result in the mother feeling less desire for sex. Many women experience increased libido when the first trimester is over. Late in pregnancy, the increasing abdominal girth may make some women physically uncomfortable. They may be more concerned about impending labor, or are just too tired for sex.

Why is My Partner Not Keen for Sex?

This could be due to the partner being worried about "hurting" the baby, or harming the pregnancy. If the pregnancy is smooth and uncomplicated, there is no scientific evidence which indicates that sex is unsafe in pregnancy. He may not be used to the physical changes which you are going through. This concern may be more pronounced nearer the end of the pregnancy for fear of hitting the engaged fetal head. It may be a wise option to avoid any intercourse during this time if it gets too uncomfortable for the both of you.

Alternatively, there are many men who feel an increase in their desire for their partner's changing bodies during pregnancy, and they may feel an increased need to express their emotions in a physical manner.

Will Sex Feel Any Different for Me?

Many pregnant women will feel that sexual intercourse is slightly better due to the increased blood flow in the pelvis, which heightens sensation and increases sensitivity. However, some will perceive this as an uncomfortable fullness in the lower abdomen. Some women may even experience womb cramps after intercourse, especially in the third trimester and this alarms them. Transient cramps after orgasms are normal, but please see your doctor should the cramps get worse in intensity or become more frequent.

The increased breast engorgement in early pregnancy may result in some tenderness should they be fondled. It may be advisable to omit this from the foreplay with your partner should this tenderness affect you.

Due to higher estrogen levels, some women experience more vaginal lubrication, which can be pleasurable for some, but increases irritation for others.

Bleeding After Sex?

If you develop any bleeding after sex, it is best to see your obstetrician. It may be normal to have a bit of spotting after sex when you are pregnant due to the increased blood flow to the genitals and cervix from the higher levels of the circulating estrogen. However, any bleeding must be fully evaluated by a

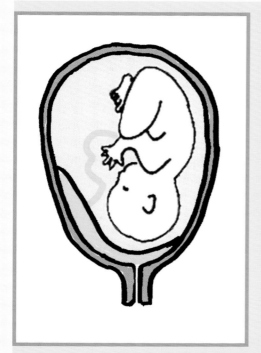

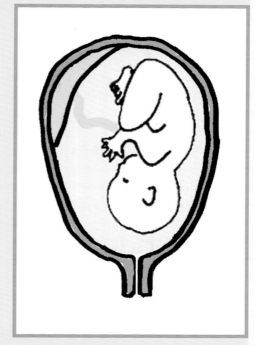

Figure19.1 Placenta Previa (arrow).   Figure 19.2 Placenta in the normal position.

simple examination and an ultrasound scan to ensure there is no serious cause for it, e.g. threatened miscarriage or preterm labor, lesions in the birth canal such as a polyp, or a low lying placenta.

When Should Sex be Definitely Avoided?

If you have **placenta previa** (a condition where the placenta lies over the internal opening of the cervix), avoid penetrative intercourse as this could result in bleeding. If your **amniotic sac has ruptured** and your waters have broken, avoid intercourse as infection could ascend to your baby. If you are in **preterm labor**, avoid intercourse as well, as orgasm and chemicals in the semen could increase uterine contractions.

You should also avoid sex in pregnancy if you have **abnormal vaginal discharge**, or if either of you has an outbreak of **herpes or any sexually transmitted infection**. Avoid sex in the third trimester if your partner had genital herpes in the past, even if he is now well and has no sores. Avoid receiving oral sex if your partner has cold sores on his mouth.

What are the Comfortable Positions for Sex?

In later pregnancy, positions like the missionary position might be difficult due to his weight on your abdomen. Deep penetration may also become more uncomfortable in the third trimester. Alternatives include lying sideways in the spoon position as this prevents deep penetration. Being on top of your partner allows you to control depth of penetration as well and keeps the weight off your abdomen. Having your partner enter you from behind while you are on all fours may also work for you. Having your partner enter you from a sitting position manages to keeps weight off your abdomen as well. Experiment with various positions till you find something that works for the both of you.

Is Oral Sex Safe in Pregnancy?

Yes, it is perfectly safe to perform oral sex on your partner. Avoid having air blown forcefully into you due to the rare possibility of an air bubble developing in a blood vessel in the area.

Are There Any Alternatives to Intercourse?

Sexual intercourse is not the only way to convey affection and desire for your partner. Some couples also engage in various other activities like hugging, kissing, massage, oral sex and masturbation.

Can Orgasms Trigger Premature Labor?

Mild cramping may follow sexual intercourse and orgasm. Orgasms cause contractions of the womb but these contractions are different from labor pains. Also, this cramping is due to the prostaglandins in semen. If your pregnancy is going well, orgasms don't lead to premature labor.

These crampings, however, should be mild and short-lived. If cramping persists or intensifies to regular contractions, you should contact your obstetrician.

Should My Partner Use a Condom?

Condoms are safe in pregnancy and prevent the transmission of sexual diseases from your partner. These diseases can affect you and your baby's health. If you have a new sexual partner during pregnancy, do consider using a condom when you have sex.

Chapter 20

Common Symptoms in Pregnancy

> *You must begin to think of yourself as becoming the person you want to be.*
>
> **David Viscott**

There are various common symptoms in pregnancy. You may or may not experience every one of them. Most of these are associated with the hormonal and physical change that accompanies each pregnancy. It is important that you are aware of these symptoms so that you will not worry unnecessarily.

Missed Periods

This is the earliest sign that you may be pregnant following conception. It is usually quite reliable especially if your periods have been regular. Bleeding may still occur if you are pregnant but it is typically lighter than your usual periods. If you have been sexually active and have missed a period, please take a urine pregnancy test.

Vaginal Bleed

At about the fifth week of pregnancy, the embryo implants itself into the lining of the womb. Some women will experience some spot-

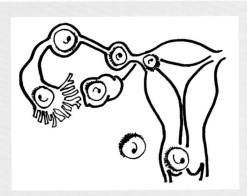

Figure 20.1 Common sites of ectopic pregnancies.

ting as well as cramping during this time. This is harmless but the bleeding may also signify other problems such as a miscarriage or an ectopic pregnancy which is a life threatening condition (whereby the pregnancy occurs outside the womb — frequently in the fallopian tubes). It is important that you seek medical advice promptly (Figures 20.1 and 20.2).

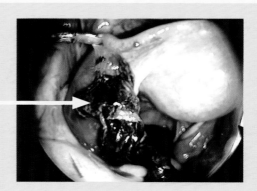

Figure 20.2 Ruptured ectopic pregnancy (arrow) in the left tube.

Breast Changes/Abdominal Bloatedness

Your breasts may become engorged and painful owing to the increase in circulating hormones. This can appear as early as a few days after conception. Throughout the pregnancy, the breast will continue to increase in size to prepare you to breastfeed the baby when it arrives. In addition, the areola (pigmented spots around the nipple) will darken.

You may even experience some tummy bloatedness as the stomach emptying slows down in pregnancy. Wearing loose clothing and eating small frequent meals may help relieve these symptoms.

Fatigue

Fatigue is also an early symptom of your pregnancy. Your body works harder to prepare itself for the next few months. It is also a way of adjusting to the emotional and physical demands. Most of the fatigue will improve as the pregnancy progresses.

Nausea/Vomiting

This is the most well-known pregnancy symptom amongst all expecting mothers. It is related to the **pregnancy hormone (Human Chorionic Gonadotrophin) which peaks at 8–10 weeks**. Rest assured that in most cases, this does not harm the developing baby — even when weight is lost in the first few months of the pregnancy. In extreme cases, anti-vomiting medications and hospitalization for intra-venous hydration may be required.

Certain conditions such as multiple pregnancies, molar pregnancies or thyroid disorders may also result in excessive vomiting, so it is important to let your doctor assess you if this happens.

Frequent Urination

The extra trips made to the toilet are most pronounced **in the early and late trimesters** of the pregnancy. Pregnancy increases your body fluids and the efficiency of your kidneys — hence the increase in urine production. In late trimesters, the additional weight of the womb on the bladder may also worsen this symptom. It is important to **exclude a urinary tract infection**, as treatment with antibiotics is required. This is usually accompanied with pain during urination. A simple urine test can be performed by your doctor to exclude an infection.

Headaches/Backaches

It is common to experience a dull backache throughout the entire pregnancy. This can worsen as the baby grows in size and weight as it adds an additional strain to your back. You may also experience headaches owing to the increase in hormonal production. **Paracetamol is safe in pregnancy** and may be used. In more severe cases, adequate bed rest and physiotherapy may be used. A referral to an orthopaedic doctor may be indicated if the backache worsens or is associated with symptoms such as sciatica — a shooting pain that runs down the back of your leg owing to nerve compression.

Food Cravings

This may become a predominant feature. Your taste buds may be numb and you may crave for sour foodstuffs. This is fine as long as you consume a healthy and well balanced diet.

Fainting Spells/Giddiness

These symptoms arise in the first 20 weeks of pregnancy as the blood pressure lowers as the blood vessels relax. Thus, if you stand for a long time or get up quickly from sitting or lying down, the flow of blood to your brain may be temporarily reduced leading to dizziness or fainting. Certain factors such as excess vomiting or heat may worsen this symptom. As your baby grows, the pressure that it exerts on your large vessels may reduce the flow of the blood to your brain further and cause more giddiness.

Certain measures may be helpful in reducing this distressing condition.

- Avoid standing for a long time.
- Getting up slowly from sitting or lying down may help in preventing a sudden reduction of blood to your brain.
- Do not go hungry.
- Do not lie flat on your back after about mid-pregnancy. It is best to lie on one side with your belly supported on a small pillow.
- If the giddiness hits you, sit or lie down.

Constipation

It is very common to become constipated while you are pregnant as food cannot move through your intestines as quickly as before. This is aggravated by your womb putting pressure on your bowels. Constipation can happen at any time during pregnancy.
To reduce this:
- Have lots of fiber, fruits and vegetables in your diet.
- Have adequate hydration.
- Exercise regularly.
- Consult your doctor if it becomes a serious problem.

Heartburn

This symptom of a burning sensation in your chest especially after meals may cause great discomfort in pregnancy. It is caused by the slowing down of your gastrointestinal tract and the relaxation of the muscles at the opening of the stomach, resulting in the reflux of the acidic gastric juices.

Certain measures may be employed to reduce this discomfort.

- Avoid food and beverages that cause heartburn.
- Take several small meals throughout the day. Also, take your time to eat and chew thoroughly.
- Try not to eat close to bedtime.
- Wear loose fitting and comfortable clothes.
- Do not lie flat on the bed. Propping yourself up against pillows may be useful.
- In more severe cases, antacids or medications may be prescribed by your doctor.

Leg Cramps

Generally, cramping of your legs begin in the second trimester and may get worse. During an attack of the cramps, **gentle stretching or massaging of the muscles** may help relieve these symptoms. It may also help to avoid sitting, standing or maintaining a fixed posture for long periods of time.

However, the cause of leg cramps is not known for certain. Some believe cramps are caused by a calcium deficiency, and that calcium tablets may help. Others believe the cramps are caused by decreased circulation of blood.

Edema or Swelling of the Legs

This is common as your body retains more fluids and your growing womb adds pressure to your legs — causing them to swell. It is worst at the end of the day especially in the third trimester. After the delivery of your baby, the swelling will disappear within weeks as your body eliminates the excess fluid through frequent urination. To minimize the swelling, it helps to put your feet up whenever you can. It is also beneficial to do gentle stretching exercises and to wear comfortable shoes.

In some cases when there is a sudden increase in leg swelling and puffiness of your face, it could be a sign of **pre-eclampsia or hypertension in pregnancy**. Consult your doctor if this happens so that your blood pressure can be monitored.

Hand Numbness

This is commonly associated with a condition known as the ***carpal tunnel syndrome***, whereby the nerve (median nerve) in the hands are compressed in a narrow space by the swelling encountered during pregnancy. Symptoms may also include tingling, burning, pain, or a dull ache in the fingers, hands or wrists. They tend to worsen in the later stage of pregnancy.

This condition tends to be worsened by repetitive hand movements. Measures that may relieve the symptoms include having a **wrist support** such as a brace and **avoiding excessive wrist flexion** in your day to day activities. **Vitamin B6** may improve the symptoms in some cases.

Hemorrhoids/Piles/Varicose Veins

These are engorged vessels that swell in the rectal area. They may cause itch, pain and bleeding when you pass motion. They occur as the enlarging womb puts pressure on the blood vessels causing them to enlarge. In most cases, they disappear after the delivery of your baby. In symptomatic cases, medications such as a topical anesthetic ointment, medicated suppositories or oral medications may be prescribed by your doctor.

For the same reason, varicosities may occur in your legs or vulva region. In cases of vulval varicosities, no treatment is needed as they will disappear after delivery. In cases of leg varicose veins, no active treatment is also required unless they give rise to symptoms such as discomfort or heaviness. Special stockings may be worn and oral medication such as Daflon may be prescribed.

Breathlessness in Pregnancy

This is a **common complaint** in pregnant mothers especially as the pregnancy advances. There is an increased need for oxygen in pregnancy, and this demand is met by your pregnancy hormones which increase your respiration. In third trimester, the enlarging womb presses onto your diaphragm and increases this sensation of breathlessness.

These symptoms are generally harmless to both you and your baby. However, there are certain medical conditions in pregnancy that may also cause breathlessness. They include a lung infection (pneumonia), asthma or pulmonary embolism — a life threatening condition whereby a blood clot goes to the lungs.

Therefore, you should seek medical attention if the breathlessness is worsening or associated with symptoms such as:
- Chest pains.
- Palpitations.
- Faintness.
- Fever.
- Cough and phlegm.

DID YOU KNOW?

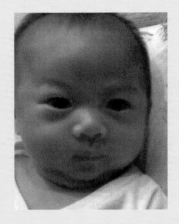

- At **28 weeks** gestation, your baby weighs an average of 1000 grams, and is about 37 cm long.
- Your baby's lungs are now mature enough to breathe air and your baby has a good chance of survival if born now.
- The eyes are also completely formed now and your baby can blink!
- Your baby may also have hiccups which you may feel as little jerks in your womb.

FREQUENTLY ASKED QUESTIONS

1. **Is it common to have nose bleeds in pregnancy?**
   Nose bleeds tend to occur more often due to the increased blood supply to the mucosa of the nose. This increased flow leads to increased pressure, which causes the delicate blood vessels to rupture. Nose bleeds are usually harmless and stop spontaneously. See your doctor if the bleed is massive.

2. **Is it common to have headaches in pregnancy?**
   Due to the increase in hormonal production, it may be common for some to experience a mild headache during pregnancy. However, ***seek immediate medical attention*** if the headaches worsen despite taking common painkillers. Other associated neurological symptoms such as vomiting, blurring of vision or weakness of the limbs may suggest more serious conditions like bleeding or tumor in the brain. Also, headaches could be a sign of an impending eclamptic fit (see Chapter 21).

3. **Is it common to have aches and pains in pregnancy?**
   During the course of your pregnancy, there is an increased elasticity of the ligaments of your birth canal to prepare you for natural vaginal delivery. However, the associated increase in motion and instability can result in pain. The affected joints commonly involve the lower back (sacro-iliac joints) and pelvis (pubic symphysis). Occasionally, as the baby grows bigger, you may even experience some discomfort in your lower rib cage.

   Aggravating factors include having a pre-existing history of low back pain or excessive physically strenuous activities during your pregnancy. Referral to an orthopedic doctor may be necessary if the backache worsens or is associated with other neurological symptoms such as sciatica which is a shooting pain that runs down the back of your leg due to nerve compression.

4. **Is it common to have bleeding in my stools?**
   It is common to experience constipation and develop piles during your pregnancy. Both conditions can have blood in your stools. Nonetheless, do inform your doctor of any bleeding especially if it is persistent so that an examination can be performed to ensure that the bleeding is not due to a more serious condition such as a cancer although this is rare in pregnancy.

5. Why is there navel (belly button) pain in pregnancy?

Belly button (umbilical) pain is common during pregnancy. Your abdominal wall is the thinnest around the navel. This increased pressure due to pregnancy may cause sensitivity and pain in this area. This is harmless and will come and go. If it keeps getting worse, or there is noticeable bulging in that area, see your doctor.

6. Why do some women experience retention of urine during pregnancy?

Retention of urine can occur at about 3 to 4 months of pregnancy in some women who have retroverted wombs which tilt backwards. So if you experience difficulty in passing urine during this period, see your doctor to exclude an urinary infection or tilted womb.

7. Is it normal to have blocked ears during pregnancy?

There are many reasons why ears are blocked during pregnancy. As a result of pregnancy changes causing swelling of the nasal lining, the tube that connects the nose to the ears (eustachian tube) may become blocked easily. Simple measures such as decongestants or nasal sprays prescribed by your doctor may be helpful. It is also important for your doctor to exclude other common conditions such as the accumulation of earwax.

If your symptoms are worsening or persistent despite the abovementioned measures, it is advisable to seek medical attention from an Ear, Nose and Throat (ENT) specialist.

Chapter 21

Pregnancy Complications

There are several medical conditions that can complicate a pregnancy. Some are more common than others. You should be aware of what these are.

First Trimester Bleeding

This is defined as vaginal bleeding or spotting that happens in the first 12 weeks of your pregnancy. Most of these bleeds are not significant and your baby is not affected in anyway. However, if persistent or associated with pain, it may indicate underlying problems such as a ***miscarriage or an ectopic pregnancy*** (pregnancy that exists outside the womb). It is imperative that you seek medical attention so that the necessary investigations can be performed.

In an ectopic pregnancy, the embryo implants into the fallopian tube after fertilization. It is more common when the fallopian tubes are damaged already. It can cause heavy internal bleeding, resulting in death. Emergency surgery may be required to treat this problem.

In most cases of early pregnancy bleeding, the baby is unaffected and the scan shows the presence of the fetal heart. In such cases of 'threatened miscarriage', the prognosis is good and usually, the baby will be fine.

Antepartum Hemorrhage (Bleeding)

This happens when the pregnant mother experiences vaginal bleeding when the baby reaches viability (> 24 completed weeks of pregnancy). In most cases, the bleeding is idiopathic, i.e. the cause is unknown and baby is usually well. It is important to rule out other more serious conditions such as a low lying placenta (placenta previa) or premature separation of the placenta from the womb (abruption placenta) (see Chapter 40 on Cesarean section).

Classically placenta previa has painless bleeds while the latter condition has painful bleeds. Both conditions can be life threatening to either the mother or the baby and may necessitate a Cesarean section as a life saving procedure. It is important to seek prompt medical attention should this symptom occur.

Pre-term Labor (PTL)

It happens when the mother experiences strong labor contractions

> **IMPORTANT!**
>
> Falls in pregnancy can cause bleeding in the placenta and preterm labor. This is especially so if there is a direct trauma to the tummy. So seek immediate medical attention if you suffer a serious fall with direct trauma to the womb.

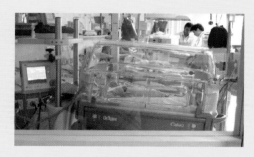

Figure 21.1: Neonatal Intensive Care Unit with premature babies in incubators.

before 37 completed weeks of pregnancy. In some cases, the symptoms may be subtle and the contractions can feel like mild menstrual cramping or backache. The risks to a premature baby include ***respiratory problems, infections, gut problems and a prolonged intensive care stay*** (Figure 21.1). All these can incur an exorbitant hospitalization bill. These risks are greater in the more premature babies (e.g. those born before 34 weeks of pregnancy). As such, hospitalization and medications such as salbutamol or nifedipine may be necessary if you experience preterm labor to help prolong the pregnancy, while steroids (dexamethasone) administered in the form of intramuscular injections to the mother help accelerate the maturity of the baby's lungs.

This condition should be clearly differentiated from Braxton-Hicks contractions — a condition characterized by irregular painless tightenings that happen from about 28 weeks of pregnancy onwards. These are harmless and will not bring about an opening of the cervix and early delivery of baby.

Pre-term Premature Rupture of Membranes (PPROM)

PPROM refers to a condition whereby the water bag that surrounds the baby in the womb leaks or ruptures before 37 weeks of pregnancy. When this happens, the risk of a pre-term delivery, infection of the mother and baby, prolapse or compression of the umbilical cord and separation of the placenta from the womb increases. You may experience a sudden gush of fluid from the vagina and the doctor can confirm this after an examination.

NOTE

If PPROM occurs **before six months of pregnancy**, the prognosis is guarded. Very often, this will lead to a spontaneous miscarriage. Even if the pregnancy continues, it may cause infection, limb contractures and poor development of the lungs (pulmonary hypoplasia), which could be fatal.

Hospitalization is required to closely monitor the expectant mother. The aim is to prolong the pregnancy for fetal maturity without compromising the mother's and the baby's well being. The mother will be closely monitored for any signs of infection such as fever, and blood tests will be performed at regular intervals.

Antibiotics will also be given to minimize the risk of an infection. Delivery will be expedited in a pre-term baby should an infection set in, or if the tests indicate that the baby is in distress inside the womb. With the right treatment, both mother and baby will be fine, although the baby may require a stay in the intensive care unit should it be born premature.

Hypertensive Disorder of Pregnancy/Pre-eclampsia

This condition is characterized by the development of high blood pressure (>140/90 mmHg), swelling of the extremities and proteins in the urine during pregnancy from >20 weeks of pregnancy onwards.

Those who are primiparas (never delivered before), above 35 years of age, with twins or triplets or have pre-existing hypertension or diabetes are at a higher risk of developing this condition. In some instances, this condition has been known to arise during labor or after the delivery of the baby. Many other organ systems can also be affected and notably seizures (eclampsia) can occur in severe cases. When the organ systems are severely affected, they can pose a danger to the mother and fetus.

Treatment entails the delivery of both the baby and the placenta.

- In *mild cases*, anti-hypertensives may be prescribed to lower the blood pressure while continuing to follow up the pregnancy closely. The baby's well being will be checked regularly through a variety of tests to ensure that it is growing properly and receiving adequate oxygen.
- In *severe cases*, admission is necessary and a medication known as Magnesium Sulphate may be administered intra-venously to prevent the mother from developing a seizure or fit.

The **warning symptoms** to this severe condition include **severe headaches, visual disturbances, severe nausea and vomiting**, and **right sided upper abdominal pain**. If you suffer from any one of these symptoms after being diagnosed with pre-eclampsia, ***prompt medical attention*** is mandatory.

Gestational Diabetes Mellitus (GDM)

Diabetes can happen in pregnancy when the body does not produce adequate amounts of the hormone **insulin** to deal with sugar control during pregnancy. As a result, the sugar levels may climb. In most cases, the condition disappears after the delivery. In others, the condition may persist and long term follow-up and treatment of the diabetes is required. A repeat **oral glucose test (OGTT)** for diabetes will be performed **six weeks after delivery**.

Testing for GDM entails drinking a sweet liquid after a night of fasting, followed by the drawing of blood samples at the onset and two hours later (oral glucose tolerance test) (see Chapter 14).

Once diagnosed, it is essential to control your blood sugar levels during the course of your pregnancy. The various measures include self-monitoring of blood glucose levels, diet and exercise management, insulin injections in more severe cases, and the close monitoring of you and your baby's well being by an experienced team of caregivers. This minimizes the risks to you and your baby. Good control means pre-meal level of 4.4–5.5 mmoL and post-meal level of 5.5–6.6 mmoL.

Untreated or poorly controlled GDM may result in fetal abnormalities, big babies (> 4 kg) causing problems during delivery, premature delivery, an increased chance of cesarean delivery and a slightly increased risk of sudden fetal death.

Group B Streptococcus (GBS) Infection

This is a type of bacterial infection that can be found in up to 30–40% of pregnant women's vagina or rectum (colonization). ***It is not a sexually transmitted disease***. The significance of this is that a small percentage of mothers can pass GBS to her baby during delivery, resulting in severe infection of the lungs and brain resulting in the possible death of the baby within the first few days of birth. A test swab of the vagina can be done at 35–37 weeks during the routine antenatal visits to **exclude** the presence of GBS colonization.

There are other symptoms that may indicate that you are at an increased risk of delivering a baby with GBS infection. These include:

- Rupture of membrane (forewaters of hindwaters) before 37 weeks or for more than 18 hours duration.
- Fever during labor (> 38°C).
- GBS urinary tract infection during your pregnancy.
- A previous baby affected with GBS infection.

If your test swab had been positive or if the above risk factors are present, your doctor will administer **_intravenous antibiotics_** during your delivery to prevent your baby from becoming infected.

Asthma in pregnancy

Asthma has been reported to affect 4%–8% of pregnant women, and is often under-recognized and sub-optimally treated. Generally, the biggest danger to the mother and her fetus comes from poorly controlled or under-treated diseases. Management during pregnancy should include education regarding use of the inhaler and reassurance about the safety of medications used to control asthma. The natural course of asthma in pregnancy is very variable and largely unpredictable. The pregnant patient and her immediate family members must be educated on their understanding of the disease, avoidance of asthma triggers, correct inhaler technique and the importance of compliance to treatment. Regular home peak flow monitoring and personalized self-management plans will prove successful in the well-motivated pregnant asthmatic.

The common warning symptoms are wheezing, shortness of breath, dry coughing, and chest tightness. Nocturnal symptoms also point to poor control of asthma, as are symptoms severe enough to affect the activities of daily living or work. Frequent usage of reliever medications, e.g. salbutamol inhalers is an important warning sign. This is especially so when the usual amount of medication is not able to provide symptomatic relief. Patients should then promptly seek the help of their doctors.

It must be emphasized that it is safer for pregnant women with asthma to be treated with asthma medications than for them to have asthmatic symptoms and complications (e.g. acute attacks which are potentially fatal in severe cases).

Pregnant women with more severe asthma have increased risks while those with better-controlled asthma are at lower risk of complications like prematurity and intra-uterine growth restriction (IUGR).

Bell's Palsy

Bell's palsy is a sudden, unilateral facial weakness without a detectable cause. It usually occurs in the age group of 15–45 years. Bell's palsy is two to three times more common in women than in men. It is three-fold more likely in pregnant than non-pregnant women. Characteristically, it occurs around term, either two weeks before or after delivery. It is present in one in 2000 pregnancies.

It has no known cause. But it is believed that Bell's palsy is caused by the inflammation of the facial nerve resulting in a one-sided weakness of the face. They may have facial drooping on the affected half. Some may even complain of excessive tear flow or a reduced sense of taste. It is important to **exclude an acute stroke, brain tumor or intracranial bleeding**.

Most patients recover without medication. 85% of patients have full recovery in 6–12 months. 10% may have partial residual facial weakness, while 5% may have severe facial weakness. Some may have reduced or loss of sense of taste permanently. The eyes are frequently unprotected in patients with Bell's palsy. This leaves the eyes at risk for corneal drying and foreign body exposure. Tear substitutes like eyedrops, lubricants, and eye protection with eye shields or glasses will be helpful.

Treatments with steroids or anti-viral medications have been used, but it is unsure if they hasten the recovery or improve the outcome of Bell's palsy.

Macrosomia (Big Baby)

This condition occurs when the birth weight of the baby is $\geq$ 4 kg. This is considerably heavier than most babies born at term. Although most of these cases have no known predisposing cause, there are a few risk factors associated with macrosomia. The more common factors include poorly controlled diabetes, those with one or more previous deliveries and those with a history of big babies in their previous pregnancies.

There are certain concerns associated with a big baby:

- The labor can be prolonged or even arrested, needing a Cesarean section.
- Delivery can be difficult and the baby's shoulder may be stuck at the birth canal (shoulder dystocia). This is an **obstetric emergency** and maneuvers will be required to deliver the baby, some of which can injure the baby or result in severe trauma to the perineum.

- There is an increased risk of baby injury from the shoulder dystocia — this can result in fractures and injuries to nerves especially to those located in the neck region (Erb's palsy).
- There is an increased risk of post delivery bleeding.
- There is an increased risk of maternal trauma from the birth process.

Intrauterine Growth Restriction (IUGR)

This is term used to describe babies who are smaller than what they should be at their gestational age. The most common cause is a problem in the placenta and this impairs the delivery of nutrition and oxygen to the baby. Smoking and excess alcohol consumption can lead to this. Birth defects and genetic disorders can also cause IUGR.

Once this problem is detected, it is essential to conduct further tests such as an ultrasound examination to measure the weight and blood flow within the baby. The amniotic fluid level (water-bag) is also assessed and the baby's heartbeat may be monitored regularly. About 60% of small babies are actually normal and are small because of their genetic make up. Just like there are different sizes of infants, children and adults, there are also different sizes of babies in the uterus.

The ultimate timing of the baby's delivery depends on how well the baby is coping inside the womb. Early delivery is only indicated if the environment inside the womb is deemed too unsafe for the baby. At times, a cesarean section may be carried out to expedite the delivery and prevent the baby from going through the stress of labor.

Abnormalities of the Amniotic Fluid Levels

1. *Oligohydramnios* (Too little fluid surrounding the baby)

The liquor in the water-bag that surrounds the baby inside the womb is maintained by the balance between the constant production of the baby's urine and the constant swallowing of the fluid by the baby. It forms a protective environment for the baby. If the amniotic fluid level is exceedingly low, it is known as oligohydramnios (usually defined as an Amniotic Fluid index of < 5). There are various reasons for this condition. They include:

- Structural defects in the baby's urinary system causing less urine production.
- Intrauterine growth retardation — where the urine production is compromised.
- Rupture of the amniotic membranes.

- Pregnancy that exceeds 42 weeks gestation (overdue babies).

The risks associated with this condition depend on the gestation and the underlying cause of the oligohydramnios. When the baby is less than 20 weeks old, this fluid is important for the structural development of the limbs and lungs. A lack of the amniotic fluid can result in limb deformities and lung underdevelopment.

The treatment for low levels of amniotic fluid is based on gestational age and underlying cause. If the baby is not full term yet, your doctor will monitor you very closely. In certain cases, a termination may be offered if the prognosis is considered very poor in those less than 24 weeks of gestation.

Further tests may be done to monitor your baby's activity. If you are close to full term, then delivery is usually recommended.

2. *Polyhydramnios* (Too much fluid surrounding the baby)

When there is an increased production of amniotic fluid, this is known as polyhydramnios. It is usually defined as an Amniotic Fluid Index (AFI) of > 25. There are numerous causes. Some of these include uncontrolled diabetes in pregnancy, fetal conditions impairing the ability to swallow and twin-to-twin transfusion in twins with a single placenta.

In addition to the problems posed by the underlying conditions, the excess fluid can cause the following:

- Pressure symptoms resulting in discomfort and breathlessness.
- Increase risk of premature labor owing to the overdistension of the womb.
- Increase risk of cord prolapse or abruptio placenta (separation of the placenta from the womb) at the time of labor.
- Increase risk of post partum hemorrhage (excessive bleeding) after the delivery of the baby.

In addition to treating the underlying cause e.g. the medical control of diabetes, amniocentesis may be performed to withdraw the excess fluid to relieve the pressure symptoms and discomfort.

Decreased Fetal Movements

You may first begin to feel your baby move at between 18–24 weeks of pregnancy. The feeling is varied and some have described it as a "wave of bubbles". This is known as **quickening**. The actual sensation of the baby's movements varies between individuals and is dependent on factors such as:

- Baby's location.
- Gestation age.
- Location of the placenta.

Therefore, although fetal movements are used as a convenient way to assess the baby's wellbeing, there can be pitfalls with this method. In general, fetal kick counts can be recorded in a fetal movement chart — registering the number and time of the kicks. It is considered normal if there are more than ten kicks over a 12-hour period. If there are few or no fetal movements felt, it is prudent to seek ***medical advice immediately***.

Overdue Babies

This happens when the pregnancies progress past the expected due date (post dates) or two weeks past the expected due dates (post term). There is a definite concern that such babies pass out meconium during labor and is associated with a higher chance of heart rate abnormalities, meconium aspiration into the lungs, cesarean sections and stillbirth. Most doctors would advocate an induction of labor to avoid these problems.

Cord Round Neck or Cord Accidents

The umbilical cord is a vital structure that delivers nutrition and oxygen to the baby. A "cord round neck" situation arises when the cord is wrapped around the baby's neck. This is usually diagnosed at the time of delivery. In most cases, this does not cause any harm to the baby, but may result in cardiotocograph abnormalities at the time of labor (known as variable decelerations). In most instances, the baby undergoes successful vaginal delivery.

On the other hand, "cord accidents" refer to a specific situation whereby problem in the cord results in the demise of the baby in-utero (stillbirth). Again, this can only be diagnosed confidently after the delivery of the stillborn, inspection of the cord and the exclusion of other causes. The cord may be found to be knotted resulting in the deprivation of oxygen to the baby (Figure 21.2). Unfortunately, there is no accurate way of diagnosing this condition antenatally.

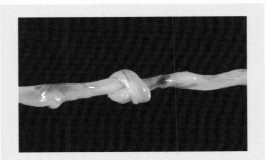

Figure 21.2 Knot in umbilical cord.

FREQUENTLY ASKED QUESTIONS

1. **Should I continue asthmatic medications during labor?**

   Acute attacks of asthma during labor and delivery are extremely rare, and women should be reassured accordingly. Regularly scheduled medications (both inhalers and even steroids) should be continued during labor. For induction of labor, the use of Prostin (Prostaglandin E2), which is a bronchodilator, is safe. Women with asthma may safely use all forms of pain relief in labor, including epidural analgesia and Entonox (see Chapter 37). If cesarean section is required, women should be encouraged to have **a regional (spinal or epidural)** rather than general anesthesia because of the increased risk of severe bronchospasm and chest infection.

2. **Are there benefits to breastfeeding for asthmatic mothers?**

   After childbirth, women with asthma should be encouraged to breastfeed. The risk of atopic disease developing in the child of an asthmatic woman is about one in 10, or one in 3 if both parents are atopic. Breastfeeding has been shown to reduce this risk. All forms of inhaled preparations and oral steroids are safe when breastfeeding.

3. **Will Hand-Foot-Mouth disease affect my pregnancy?**

   Hand, foot and mouth disease (HFMD) is a virus usually caused by the **Coxsackie A virus**. It is infectious and spreads through coughs, sneezes and contact with feces. It is common in children but rare in healthy adults.

   The early symptoms are fever and sore throat, followed by sores in the mouth and on the hands and feet. The incubation period (time between catching the disease and showing symptoms) is 3–6 days — during which time the virus can be passed on. Treatment is aimed at relieving symptoms. **There is normally no risk to your baby.** However, any viral infections, if serious enough may cause miscarriages although this is very rare.

   The risk to your baby increases if you catch the virus shortly before delivery. Your baby may be infected and may need hospital treatment to avoid further problems.

4. **Should I induce my labor if my baby is "biggish"?**

   Routine induction of labor is commonly practiced but this has not been found to conclusively improve outcomes for both the mother and baby.

Moreover, ultrasound estimation of the baby's weight is *not 100% accurate*, with measurement error of 20%. On the other hand, routine cesarean sections, with their associated surgical risks, have never been proven to reduce morbidity in babies except in some cases associated with diabetes.

5. Is it normal to salivate more during my pregnancy?

It can happen to some women during their pregnancy. There may be various reasons why this arises. Changing hormonal levels during the pregnancy may contribute to increased salivation.

Morning sickness causing nausea can also lead to increased production of saliva. Heartburn, resulting from the acidic contents of your stomach, may irritate your salivary glands and worsen this problem. In these situations, over the counter medications (e.g. antacids) can be used to help reduce the salivation.

6. Is "trigger finger" more common during pregnancy?

This is a condition characterized by discomfort in the palm during movement of the involved fingers. In some cases, the tendon causes a painful click as the patient flexes and extends the finger. The finger may even be locked in a particular position, usually in flexion, which may need gentle passive manipulation. The problem results from inflammation of tendons located within a protective covering called the tendon sheath.

Common causes include repetitive usage of the fingers. It is also associated with medical conditions like diabetes and autoimmune diseases. There is no association with pregnancy. It is important to see a doctor. Treatment can range from simple pain-killers, splinting to local injections.

7. My heart is beating at a faster rate since pregnancy. Is this normal?

It is part of the body's normal physiological response to pregnancy. This is to cope with the demands of increased blood supply to the baby via the placenta. However, if you start experiencing chest pains as well as shortness of breath even at rest, please see your doctor immediately to exclude heart problems.

8. **What happens if I have dengue fever during pregnancy? Will my baby be affected?**

Dengue is a mosquito-borne virus infection and is endemic in Southeast Asia. It causes myalgia, high fever and a drop in the blood platelet level with bleeding tendencies. There have been no reports of teratogenic effect of the dengue virus causing fetal malformations in the first and second trimesters.

Although rare, there have been reports of vertical transmission from the mother to the baby. Those cases occurred at or near the time of delivery. As a result, the affected infants can develop a fever as well as bleeding tendencies due to low platelet levels.

Chapter 22

Twin Pregnancy — Double Joy or Double Trouble?

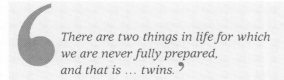

> There are two things in life for which
> we are never fully prepared,
> and that is … twins.
>
> **Josh Billings**

You are unique if you are carrying twins! Twins occur only in *one in every 80 pregnancies*. There are many unique issues in twin pregnancies, which you will need to understand.

Identical and Non-identical Twins

One third of twins are identical and two-thirds non-identical.

In **identical (monozygotic) twins**, one egg is fertilized by one single sperm, but the egg divides into two embryos soon afterwards. Thus, both twins have the same genetic material and will have the same sex with perfect resemblance.

The **identical twins** can share one placenta ("mono-chorionic") or have two different placentas ("di-chorionic"). They can be housed in one water sac ("mono-amniotic") or two separate water-sacs ("di-amniotic") (Figures 22.1 and 22.2).

It is important to know whether the twins are identical

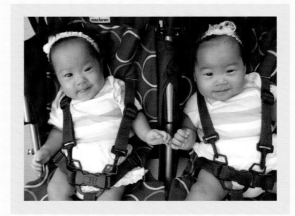

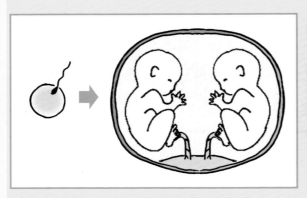
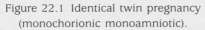
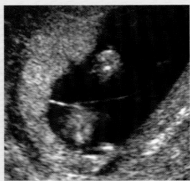

Figure 22.1 Identical twin pregnancy (monochorionic monoamniotic).

Figure 22.2 Ultrasound scan of monochorionic diamniotic twins.

or non-identical as identical twins have increased risks, which will be described later. **This check for chorionicity is best done by ultrasound scan in the first trimester**.

On the other hand, **non-identical (dizygotic) twins** occur when two separate eggs are fertilized by two separate sperms. Thus, the genetic make-ups of both twins are different and they can be of the same sex or different sex. Each twin will have its own water sac and placenta (Figure 22.3).

Possible Problems of Twin Pregnancies

While it is a great joy to carry twins, *more complications may arise* as compared to a singleton (one baby) pregnancy.

Mothers who are carrying twins tend to get high blood pressure and diabetes in pregnancy more commonly. They are also prone to anemia and thus need iron supplementation.

There is an increased risk of miscarriage in twins during early pregnancy. Unfortunately, miscarriage of one twin can sometimes occur. If this occurs early in the pregnancy, the mother's body will simply absorb the remaining tissue. If it happens late in the pregnancy, very close observation and follow-up is required. The remaining twin may suffer from mental handicap from the toxins released due to the dead twin, especially if they share a common placenta.

Down syndrome screening test is best done by a **nuchal translucency (neck thickness) scan** of both twins at 12–13 weeks.

Preterm delivery is common in twin pregnancy, usually before 36 weeks instead of 40 weeks as in singleton pregnancy. However, premature delivery can occur as early as 6–7 months of pregnancy. The babies may not survive at

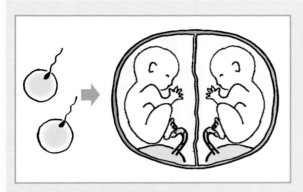

Figure 22.3 Non identical twin pregnancy (dichorionic diamniotic).

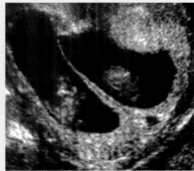

Figure 22.4 Ultrasound scan of di-amniotic dichorionic twins.

such prematurity and may need prolonged stay in the neonatal intensive care unit. **Identical twins are usually delivered earlier at around 34–36 weeks.**

The growth of both twins will need close monitoring, especially in identical twins. Your doctor will see you more frequently during your pregnancy as compared to a singleton pregnancy. Ultrasound sessions would be done more frequently to chart the progress of the growth of both babies.

Monochorionic twins who share a single placenta may not share the blood flow in the placenta equally. This leads to "twin–twin transfusion" and may occur in 15% of such pregnancies. Most cases are mild. However, serious cases can be dangerous to both babies and will require a specialist's management.

Problems with Triplets and Higher-Order Mutiple Pregnancies

The chance of spontaneous triplet and higher-order multiple pregnancies is rare. However, with in vitro-fertilization (test-tube babies) and other assisted reproductive programs, these pregnancies can happen more often.

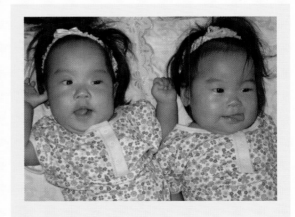

Your doctor will need to discuss the risks of triplet pregnancies carefully. All the risks discussed above are mutiplied many fold. The risk of preterm delivery is extremely high and most triplets deliver at about 7–8 months. They will usually need to stay in the neonatal intensive care unit after delivery because of low birth weight and prematurity.

Social Implications of a Twin Pregnancy

Very clearly, there are direct financial implications when the twins are due. You will need to buy two of everything. You will need double sized push-chairs, need to double up on the supplies, have double food to buy, need two car seats, etc.

Other than the stress of financial support, you will need to cope with double the number of nappies to change, twice the crying (in volume or in duration) and double the late night wake up calls. You will definitely need more help!

However, there are upsides too. After all, if you were planning to have two kids only, then you have to go through the pregnancy process only once. Thus, although there could be double trouble, there is double joy as well!

DID YOU KNOW?

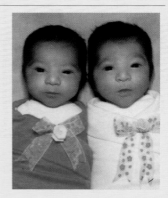

- At **32 weeks** gestation, baby is an average of 2000 grams and is about 42 cm long.
- Your baby's five senses are now developed and functioning. Your baby can also see light through the womb and react to it.
- Your baby can now also produce tears.
- Your baby develops rapid eye movements (REM) sleep now and is capable of dreams!

Chapter 23

Vaginal Discharge During Pregnancy

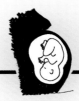

> *What's that on the telly?*
> *It's an angel sent from God...*
> *Growing in my belly...*
> *Like a sweet pea in a pod!*
>
> **Melissa Hatcher**

Most women would notice an increase in vaginal discharge during pregnancy. This is quite normal and is caused by a combination of factors — increased blood supply, softening of the cervix and vaginal walls, and later, stimulation from the baby's head, as he or she presses against the cervix ready for labor.

Normal vaginal discharge is clear, white or creamy, and fairly runny. It may have a distinctive odor, but not an unpleasant smell. **Signs of infection** include thick, curd-like or greenish discharge, a nasty smell, itchy and soreness, low abdominal pain or pain during sex.

When you are about to go into labor, your discharge may contain streaks of thick mucus and a little fresh blood, as the cervical mucus plug is dislodged from the cervix. This is known as **the show**. Having a show does not necessarily mean that labor is about to start, but it is a reasonable indication that the cervix is beginning to ripen or to prepare for labor. Some women have shows off-and-on for several days before the actual labor.

What Can I Do About It?

An increase in vaginal discharge is a normal part of pregnancy. Remind yourself that this discharge plays a part in protecting your uterus from infection ascending up the vagina. However, be aware of changes to your discharge, and highlight this to your doctor if you think things may not be quite right. Your doctor may take a **vaginal swab** to check for an infection such as **candidiasis, Group B streptococcus (GBS) or gardnerella**. The result of this should be known within one week. Most vaginal infections can be effectively treated during pregnancy.

Proper hygiene and, if necessary, the use of panty liners should keep you feeling fresh. Avoid excessive vaginal douches and scented hygiene wipes — as they may cause irritation and may upset the delicate acid/alkali balance of the vagina.

Common Vaginal Infections in Pregnancy

1. Vaginal candidiasis (moniliasis or thrush)

This is a common and frequently distressing fungal infection for many women during pregnancy. It does not harm the baby during pregnancy or childbirth. Having vaginal thrush can cause extreme itch and clumps of white discharge. Because of the hormonal changes, pregnant women often get thrush, especially during the third trimester of pregnancy. Fortunately, it does not cause the baby any harm and can be easily treated by vaginal pessaries and cream. It may recur throughout pregnancy but usually has no long standing effects on the pregnancy.

2. Group B streptococcal infection (GBS)

Group B streptococcus is a type of bacteria found in the vagina and rectum in about 30–40% of women (see Chapter 21). Late in your third trimester you may be tested for GBS. Testing involves inserting a cotton swab into the vagina. The swab is then sent to the laboratory to see if this particular bacteria is present. If it is present, you will require **intravenous antibiotics** during labor to reduce the risk of infection in the baby.

3. Gardnerella infection (bacterial vaginosis)

This is a type of bacteria that is usually found in the vagina but is kept under control by the presence of other types of harmless bacteria that produce chemicals to keep the vagina slightly acidic. Bacterial vaginosis, caused by the overgrowth of these bacteria, can cause abnormal vaginal odor and discharge. It is common in pregnancy and has been found to be associated with a higher risk of preterm delivery and rupture of the membranes. This can be easily treated with antibiotics, either orally or inserted into the vagina.

4. *Vaginal bleeding*

If you have bleeding from your vagina, put on a sanitary pad and observe its amount. Many women lose a small amount of blood at some point in their pregnancy and, often, this is of little significance. However, occasionally, vaginal bleeding may indicate a serious problem — a threatened miscarriage, a low-lying placenta or a polyp in the cervix — so it is always best to get advice from a doctor.

It is wise to note the following:

- The color of the blood (dark or bright red).
- The quantity (just a smear, a teaspoon, a tablespoon, or soaking through pads and clothing).
- The presence or absence of pain (continual, cramping, contractions and so on).
- Whether you had sex recently.
- The frequency of your baby's movements (often a useful clue to his or her wellbeing).
- Your pregnancy details so far (including the results of any ultrasound scans).

How to Differentiate between Vaginal Discharge, Urine or Bleeding?

It may be difficult at times to differentiate these symptoms. If you are unsure whether you have a heavy vaginal discharge, stress urinary incontinence, or are leaking amniotic fluid, put on a sanitary pad to check on the discharge. Consult your doctor as soon as you can.

Chapter 24

Pregnancy Loss and Ways to Cope

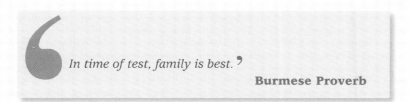

In time of test, family is best.

Burmese Proverb

Losing your baby early in pregnancy, later on during delivery or after birth is an event which has potential immense psychological impact on you and your partner's life.

Early Pregnancy Loss

About 20% of women suffer from a miscarriage early in pregnancy (usually up to 12 weeks gestation), and in the majority of women, **the cause is not known**. A miscarriage often brings about despair, depression and shock to the parents. This effect is more pronounced, especially if there had been a history of infertility or previous pregnancy losses. Other causes of early pregnancy loss include chromosomal or genetic defects in the fetus, which by natural selection, will not be sustained. In most pregnancies, the event is only a sporadic one and therefore, will not affect the chance of success in subsequent pregnancies. It is only when miscarriages happen for **three or more times (recurrent miscarriages)**, that we would be concerned about underlying defects in the parents. Under these circumstances, a more thorough assessment and investigation of the couple is warranted.

Late Pregnancy Loss/Intrauterine Death

Stillbirth is an unforeseen event and is defined by the death of a baby when it is **born after 24 weeks of pregnancy**. Fortunately this occurs only in 1:100–200 pregnancies, but when it happens, it is devastating. In many cases the cause of death of the baby cannot be established and there is no way of reliably predicting its occurrence during the antenatal period. Other known causes include placental problems, growth restriction of the baby, infections, birth defects, umbilical cord accidents, chronic maternal diseases (such as diabetes, high blood pressure), post term pregnancy (>42 weeks of pregnancy) and Rhesus incompatibility.

Will Induction of Labor be Necessary?

Some women will find it very difficult to come to terms with the fact that they are still carrying a fetus that is no longer alive in their womb. Studies have shown that a woman is much more likely to suffer from depressive symptoms after delayed delivery of a stillborn of more than three days. Most women will opt for an induction of labor to avoid this. The doctor may take into account the mental state, physical conditions and advise on when is the best time to induce delivery. The aim ultimately is to allow for a vaginal delivery. This avoids having to put the mum through the risks associated with a cesarean section.

On the other hand, it is **generally safe to delay delivery** and await spontaneous labor provided there are no other conditions such as:

- A rupture of membranes predisposing to infection in the womb.
- Severe medical conditions like uncontrolled diabetes or hypertension.
- Abruptio placenta which is a life-threatening condition resulting from the placental separation from the womb.

There is also a theoretical concern that clotting problems may develop in the body as delivery is delayed for a long period of time (> 4 weeks). As such, periodic blood tests to screen for such clotting problems may be necessary if delivery is still delayed after a few weeks.

Is There Help Available?

It is perfectly normal to grieve over your pregnancy loss. The grief process goes through the different phases of **denial, bargaining, anger, sadness** and then finally **acceptance** of the situation. In fact, you should start to feel gradually better as time passes. Seek professional help if you find great difficulty in overcoming the grief and you are not able to cope with everyday life. Most people who suffer loss of loved ones go through a process of grief reaction which eventually leads them to emotional healing. The feelings you may experience may include shock and denial, guilt and anger, depression and despair, and finally acceptance.

Finding a way to manage your grief may aid in your recovery process. You might consider holding a small memorial service, or a symbolic ceremony to share your thoughts about your baby. You may also want to share your thoughts through a **support group** with others who have experienced pregnancy losses. Your doctor may encourage you and your family members to see, hold and touch your baby, although this may be a very difficult and painful moment. Even if there is some malformation of the baby, seeing is better as what is often imagined by the woman is often worse than reality. Holding and giving your baby a name may aid in your recovery process. You may want to save a photo or other momentos which you can cherish when you think about your lost baby.

In KK hospital, a mental wellness service has been set up to help grieving mothers cope with their pregnancy loss better. Comprising of a psychiatrist, psychologist and a medical social worker, it aims to provide a holistic approach to grieving mothers. There is even a support group known as the Perinatal Depression and Anxiety Support and Education Group set up. More information can be obtained through our hotline at (+652) 6394 3739.

In addition to the above-mentioned emotional aspects, some other medical issues need to be addressed as well. They include:

- **Suppression of lactation** to avoid breast engorement and discomfort. This can be achieved by cold cabbage treatment, a good supportive bra and pain-killers. If necessary, specific medicines may be prescribed (Dostinex or Cabergolin).
- **Contraceptive methods** must be discussed as it is still possible to get pregnant before the first period. Pregnancy that occurs too soon may be detrimental and you should try to conceive again after the grieving process is over.

Why Did It Happen?

The painful question of "WHY" this has happened may or may not be answered. Often no specific cause is recognized as the baby looks normal. The only way to uncover reasons for the demise is to examine the pregnancy history, perform a series of blood investigations on the mother and to perform a detailed and complete examination of the fetus (postmortem). **Postmortem examination** may provide the reason for the baby's demise. Contrary to what most people think, a postmortem examination is conducted with utmost respect to the baby by a fully trained and qualified doctor. This procedure does not mutilate the body which can then be returned intact to the parents.

Knowing what happened need not tell why it had happened in the first place, but it puts a closure to the event. In instances that a cause is found, possible interventions or treatment may be administered in subsequent pregnancies to help manage it better.

Chapter 25

Nutrition During Pregnancy — Eating Right for Two

> *Proper diet can become an instrument for maintaining health and cultivating increased levels of awareness.*
> **Qigong Master Mantak Chia**

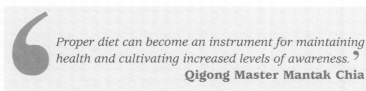

Eating healthy before conception and throughout pregnancy is one of the best things you can do for yourself and your baby. Good nutrition optimizes the growth and development of your baby and safeguards your own health.

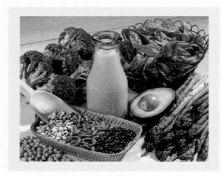

During pregnancy, your energy requirement increases by about 300 kcal a day, which is not much compared to the average non-pregnant Singapore woman's requirement of 1700 kcal a day. On the other hand, requirements for other nutrients (e.g. protein, folate, calcium, vitamin D and B vitamins) may be significantly higher than in the non-pregnancy state. As such, you should make smart choices by choosing a variety of nutrient-dense foods, rather than just eating more food! This is especially so if you now experiencing a smaller appetite.

Essential Nutrients for Pregnancy

More than 40 different types of nutrients are needed to sustain good health and promote your unborn child's growth and development. Yet, certain nutrients are especially important to ensure optimal pregnancy outcomes.

1. Folate (also known as folic acid)

Folate is vitamin B, which is essential for cell division and organ formation. This nutrient helps **prevent neural tube defects** (malformations of the brain and spinal cord) in your developing baby and **anemia** in pregnant woman. Due to the severe nature of neural tube defects, we strongly advise adequate folate intake of at least 800 micrograms daily before conception and throughout the first three months of pregnancy.

Dark green vegetables, for example, spinach, broccoli and asparagus; citrus fruits and juices, yeast extract, liver, dried beans and fortified breakfast cereals — are rich in folate. Care should be taken, however, to avoid overcooking the vegetables as folate is easily destroyed by heat.

2. Iron

Iron is needed for the formation of red blood cells. Inadequate iron intake may lead to anemia. This is because, during pregnancy, your blood volume expands to accommodate the changes in your body. Moreover, your unborn baby also needs to store adequate iron for the first six months of life before he/she starts consuming solid foods.

There are two forms of iron in foods — heme and non-heme. Heme iron is better absorbed by the body than non-heme iron. Sources of **heme iron** include red meat, liver, chicken and fish. Sources of **non-heme iron** include egg yolk, green leafy vegetables, iron-fortified breakfast cereals, dried fruits and nuts.

To enhance the absorption of non-heme iron, **consume vitamin C-rich foods** (namely, fruits and vegetables) at the same meal or take vitamin C supplements.

3. Vitamin B12

This vitamin is required for blood formation. It is only found in foods of animal origin, namely, meat, poultry, fish, milk and eggs. Vegans (vegetarians who do not eat any animal products including eggs and milk) must take vitamin B12 supplements in order to meet the daily requirements.

4. Omega-3 Fatty Acids

DHA (Docosahexaenoic acid), one of the omega-3 fatty acids, found in coldwater deep-sea fish, is important for brain and eye development. Studies have shown that pregnant women who eat cold-

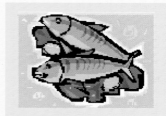

water fish have babies with higher IQ and better vision than pregnant women who do not.

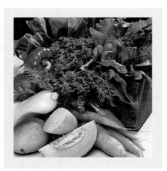

Unfortunately, large deep-sea fishes may contain methylmercury, a heavy metal that is toxic to the developing fetus's neurological system. Hence, the US Food and Drug Administration recommends that pregnant women eat a maximum of 12 ounces (3 servings) of a variety of cooked fish or shellfish per week, and *avoid shark, swordfish, king mackerel (known as "batang fish" locally) and tilefish (also called white snapper).* Although tuna is a good source of DHA, albacore tuna (found mainly as canned white tuna) is higher in methylmercury than other types of tuna (e.g. skipjack, bigeye and yellowfin, commonly used for canned light tuna), hence pregnant women are also advised to limit albacore tuna to one serving a week. **Safe DHA-rich sources** *include salmon, sardines, herring, halibut,. canned light tuna and omega-3 fortified eggs.* Alternatively, you can ask your doctor to recommend a suitable DHA supplement (300 mg a day) (see Chapter 27).

5. Vitamin A

The function of vitamin A is to promote growth of cells and tissues, and prevent night blindness. However, **excessive intake** of vitamin A above 10,000 IU daily in the first trimester can **cause birth defects**. Hence, in the first trimester, pregnant women should obtain their vitamin A from food rather than from supplements, and limit liver intake to two tablespoons (50 g) per week. **Good sources** include eggs, milk, deep-red and yellow fruits and vegetables (for example, papaya, mango, pumpkin, carrots) and dark-green leafy vegetables (for example, spinach and broccoli).

6. Calcium

Both you and your baby need calcium for strong bones and teeth. Excellent sources of calcium are milk, cheese and yoghurt. Other foods that contain calcium are beancurd ("tauhu" and "tawkwa"), green leafy vegetables, ladies fingers, small fish with edible bones such as *"ikan bilis"* and sardines, and calcium-fortified soymilk and fruit juice.

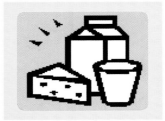

If you have lactose intolerance (i.e. bloatedness, wind, diarrhoea after drinking milk), you can consume low-lactose or lactose-free milk, calcium-fortified soymilk, cheese or yoghurt as alternatives to milk. Your doctor can also prescribe a calcium supplement (Table 25.1).

Table 25.1 Recommended daily dietary intake of calcium.

Groups	Recommended daily intake (mg/day)
Pregnant women	1000
Breastfeeding mothers	1000

Source: National Academy of Science 2000.

7. Vitamin C

Vitamin C is required for collagen formation in bones, muscles and blood vessels. The **Singapore RDA for vitamin C intake in pregnancy is 50 mg a day**, whilst the US recommendation is 85 mg a day. It is recommended that pregnant women obtain their vitamin C from food rather than from supplements, as there have been reports of rare cases of 'rebound scurvy' occurring in infants born to mothers taking 400 mg or more of vitamin C throughout their pregnancy. "Rebound scurvy" occurs when the infant becomes tolerant to the high dose of vitamin C from the mother during pregnancy, hence it develops symptoms of scurvy or vitamin C deficiency after birth.

Both our Healthy Diet Pyramid for Pregnancy and the Health Promotion Board's Healthy Diet Pyramid for Adults recommend two servings each of fruits and vegetables, which can meet the pregnancy requirements (Table 25.2). In

Table 25.2 Vitamin C content per serving of some local fruits and vegetables.

Fruit/Vegetable	Vitamin C (mg)
Papaya, 1 wedge	93
Orange, 1 small	88
Watermelon, 1 slice	11
Banana, 1 medium	8
Yellow Pear, 1 small	6
Apple, 1 small	6
Broccoli, cooked, ¾ mug	65
Cauliflower, cooked, ¾ mug	44
Cabbage, cooked, ¾ mug	20
Lady's finger, cooked, 100g	16
Spinach, cooked, ¾ mug	10

general, all types of fruits and vegetables are safe if consumed in moderation.

8. *Vitamin D*

Vitamin D helps with calcium absorption. **Food sources** include fortified milk, margarine and cold water deep-sea fishes, e.g. salmon and sardines. Apart from foods, our bodies can also synthesize vitamin D when exposed to sunlight. Spending 10 to 15 minutes twice a week outdoors is

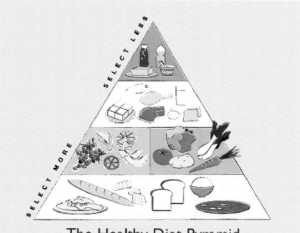

The Healthy Diet Pyramid

Figure 25.1 The healthy diet pyramid for pregnancy.

DID YOU KNOW?

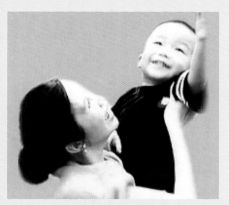

- At **36 weeks** gestation, your baby will weigh an average of 2500 grams and is 47 cm long.
- Most of your baby's basic physical maturation is complete, and your baby will spend the next few weeks putting on weight.

sufficient for our bodies to synthesize enough vitamin D to meet our requirements.

What to Eat and How Much?

The Healthy Diet Pyramid for Pregnancy is a useful guide for pregnant women to plan out their daily diet. It enables you to obtain all the important nutrients required to support a healthy pregnancy. Figure 25.1 provides more information on how to use the healthy diet pyramid.

At the tip of the pyramid are fats, oils, sugar and salt. Use in small amounts to enhance the flavour of foods.

Table 25.3 Recommended daily servings and serving sizes for the 4 food groups.

Food groups	Nutrients provided	Recommended servings per day	Examples of one serving
Rice and alternatives	• Carbohydrates, your body's preferred source of energy. • Wholegrain and enriched products contain fiber, B vitamins, various minerals and protein. • Fortified cereals provide iron and folate.	6 to 7	½ bowl of rice or noodles 2 slices bread 2 small chapati 1 piece thosai 1 hotdog bun 4 plain biscuits 1 cup breakfast cereal
Fruits	Vitamins, minerals, fiber and phytochemicals.	2	1 small apple/pear/orange 1 medium banana 1 wedge papaya/pineapple /watermelon/honeydew 6 rambutans/duku/lychees 10 grapes ¼ cup dried fruit
Vegetables	Vitamins, minerals, fiber and phytochemicals. Dark green vegetables are rich in vitamin A, iron and folate.	2 (including 1 serving of green leafy vegetables)	¾ mug* (100 g) of cooked vegetables * refers to 250 ml mug
Meat and alternatives	Protein, B vitamins and iron.	2	1 palm-sized piece of meat/fish/poultry 5 medium prawns 2 small sotong/cuttlefish/ squid 2 small squares of beancurd ¾ cup of cooked lentils, peas, beans
Milk and dairy products	Protein, calcium, phosphorus, vitamins A and D	2 to 4	1 glass milk/high-calcium soymilk 2 slices cheese 1 cup yoghurt

Foods to Avoid

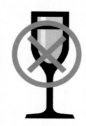

Food safety is extremely important during pregnancy. This is because bacterial toxins and certain harmful chemicals such as alcohol and methylmercury can pass from mother to baby, and cause undesirable outcomes.

The list below shows the foods to be avoided:

Unpasteurized milk; soft cheeses, e.g. Brie, feta, Camembert and Roquefort; liver pates; and uncooked hot dogs, ham and luncheon meats
These foods are prone to *Listeria monocytogenes*, a bacteria that causes listeriosis, which may result in miscarriages and stillbirth.

Raw or undercooked meat, poultry, seafood, e.g. raw oyster, cockles, sashimi and sushi; and raw or half-boiled eggs

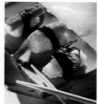

Raw and undercooked animal foods contain a variety of food-borne bacteria and viruses. Changes in your metabolism and circulation during pregnancy may increase the risk of bacterial food poisoning, and your reaction may be more severe than if you were not pregnant. Avoid raw or half-boiled eggs.

Avoid swordfish, shark, tilefish and king mackerel. Limit canned albacore tuna.

Herbal supplements

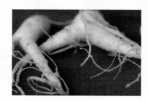

Herbal products have not been studied enough to be recommended during pregnancy. Do consult you doctor if you are planning to take these herbs (see Chapter 26).

Alcohol
Mothers who drink alcohol have a higher risk of miscarriages and stillbirth, and excessive alcohol consumption may result in fetal alcohol syndrome, including facial deformities, low birth weight and mental retardation.

Unwashed salad and raw vegetables sprouts, including alfalfa, clover, radish, and mung bean
Unwashed salads may be contaminated with bacteria from the soil, while raw vegetables sprouts contain high levels of germs, which can be harmful to health.

Healthy Weight Gain during Pregnancy

As a general guide, you can use your rate of weight gain as an indicator of whether you are eating enough for both yourself and your baby. Gaining the appropriate amount of weight in pregnancy ensures that your baby is of good birth-weight and also means that you do not have too many extra kilos to shed after delivery.

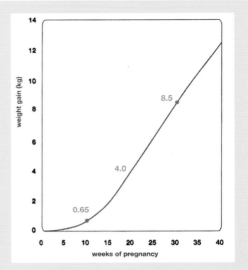

Figure 25.2 Recommended average weight gain during pregnancy.

How much weight you need to gain depends on various factors including your pre-pregnancy weight, your health status and whether you are carrying a single baby or twins/triplets. You can discuss with your doctor to determine how much weight you should gain. Most pregnant women should expect a **weight gain of 10–12 kg** throughout the entire pregnancy.

The weight gain of the mother is mainly due to the increased water retention, thus, maternal weight gain **does not necessarily correlate** well with the baby's weight at delivery.

If you are carrying twins or triplets, you will need to gain more weight. Work with your doctor to determine how much weight you should put on.

If you have gained more weight than recommended, do not try to lose weight. It is never safe to lose weight during pregnancy as both you and your baby need nutrients for growth and optimal health. You may aim for a slower rate of weight gain. Work with your doctor or request for a **referral to a dietitian** to plan out a suitable meal plan.

Special Diets

1. If you are diabetic during pregnancy

Diabetes during pregnancy increases the risk of certain health problems like high blood pressure during pregnancy (pre-eclampsia), big baby leading to difficult delivery and higher chance of needing a cesarean section. Hence, it is important for women with pre-existing diabetes before pregnancy, and those newly diagnosed during pregnancy (i.e. gestational diabetes) to control their blood glucose levels. This will minimize the risk of developing these problems.

There are three steps to manage diabetes during pregnancy, namely, *blood glucose monitoring, diet and insulin* (if blood glucose levels cannot be controlled by diet alone). Apart from controlling blood glucose levels, the diet should also provide adequate nutrition for the pregnant mother and her baby, resulting in appropriate weight gain similar to that for non-diabetic women.

The diet for diabetes during pregnancy is similar to the healthy diet recommended for all pregnant women, except for the regular distribution and consistent intake of carbohydrate-containing foods (e.g. rice and alternatives, starchy vegetables, fruits and milk) throughout the day. In other words, having **three meals and three snacks**, with the same amount of carbohydrate-containing foods daily at each meal and snack. Contrary to popular belief, there is no need for pregnant women to consume glucose or any other sugars for energy, as carbohydrate foods are digested into glucose by the body. Hence, **sugars and sweet foods are not recommended for pregnant women with diabetes**, as they are high in carbohydrates, leading to high blood glucose levels, which are often low in nutrients and high in energy, leading to excessive weight gain.

The guidelines for the diet for diabetes during pregnancy can be summarized in Table 25.4. Please see your dietitian for a meal plan specific to your needs.

2. If you have high blood pressure during pregnancy

In those suffering from long standing essential hypertension (even before pregnancy), antihypertensive medications and a low-salt diet is advocated to help treat this condition.

In hypertension that arises only during the course of the pregnancy (gestational hypertension or preeclampsia), the only definative cure for this condition is through the delivery of the baby and the placenta (see Chapter 21). However, while not a cure for pre-eclampsia, **limiting salt intake** is advised.

3. If you have phenylketonuria (PKU)

People with PKU have a **deficiency of an enzyme**, which is necessary for the proper metabolism of an amino acid called phenylalanine. Serum phenylalnine level at conception is critical to the organ development of the fetus. Elevated maternal blood levels of phenylalnine may cause **spontaneous abortion, brain and heart defects, poor fetal growth, as well as mental retardation in the baby**. If maternal blood levels of phenylalnine are optimized by special diet prior to conception and during pregnancy, this risk to the fetus is markedly

Table 25.4 Diabetic diet recommendations.

Eat Freely — foods which do not contain significant amounts of carbohydrates or energy	Eat in Controlled Amounts (as specified in your meal plan) — foods which contain carbohydrates	Eat in Moderation (as specified in your meal plan) — foods which contain energy. Can lead to becoming overweight during pregnancy if eaten in excessive amounts	Restrict (unless specified in your meal plan)
Non-starchy vegetables, e.g. green leafy vegetables, tomatoes, cucumber, mushrooms, lady's fingers.	Rice and alternatives, e.g. rice, noodles, bread, cereals, crackers.	Meat and alternatives, e.g. lean meat, chicken without skin, fish, eggs, tauhu, taukwa.	Sugars and sweet foods, e.g. table sugar, brown sugar, jam, honey, fruit juice, tinned fruit, sweet drinks, cakes, sweet pastries, desserts, chocolate, sweets.
Unsweetened beverages, e.g. water, non-cream soups, unsweetened chrysanthemum tea.	Starchy vegetables, e.g. potato, sweet potato, yam, tapioca, pumpkin, sweetcorn.		Fats and oils, e.g. fried foods, foods cooked with coconut milk or cream, nuts, salad dressings.
Seasonings & non-sweet sauces, e.g. soy sauce, curry powder, herbs and spices, pepper, vinegar.	Pulses and beans, e.g. dahl, baked beans, red beans, green beans.		Limit sweet sauces like tomato ketchup and chilli sauce to 2 teaspoons a day.
	Fresh fruits, e.g. apple, pear, honeydew, papaya, grapes, banana.		Consume artificial sweeteners and artificially-sweetened drinks and foods in small amounts (e.g. two packets sweetener or one can of artificially-sweetened drink).
	Milk & dairy products, e.g. skimmed milk, plain yoghurt.		Limit plain tea and coffee to two cups a day to prevent excessive caffeine intake.

reduced. It is important for any woman with PKU who is contemplating pregnancy to understand this.

4. If you are underweight during pregnancy

If you are underweight before pregnancy, or not putting on enough weight during pregnancy, you can still follow the Healthy Diet Pyramid for Pregnancy. Increase the number of servings consumed from each food group. If you are unable to eat more food, you can also increase your weight by:

- Snacking on healthy snacks like nuts, dried fruits, cheese, desserts (tauhuay, tauswan, red bean soup) in between meals.
- Drinking 1–2 cups of soybean milk, fruit juice, malted milk drinks (e.g. Milo, Ovaltine, Horlicks), place of plain water.
- Frying your foods in mono or polyunsaturated oils (e.g. olive, canola, sunflower, soybean oils) to increase energy intake from good fats.
- Drinking nutritional supplement drinks formulated for weight gain (e.g. Ensure, Nutren Optimum, Enercal Plus, Resource, Fortijuice).

Please discuss with your doctor if you have concerns about your weight.

5. If you are overweight during pregnancy

If you are over-weight in pregnancy or have put on too much weight during pregnancy, there is higher **risk of developing diabetes during pregnancy**. Moreover, you may find it more difficult to lose the extra weight after delivery. Thus, it increases the risk of obesity-related conditions like high blood pressure, diabetes or heart disease.

Follow the Healthy Diet Pyramid for Pregnancy, but control the number of servings consumed from each food group to the lower end of the recommended range, i.e. consume six servings of rice and alternatives, and two servings of milk and dairy products.

If you are still putting on too much weight,

- **Limit your fat intake** by cutting down on high fat foods, e.g. fried foods, foods cooked with coconut milk, nuts, fast foods, cakes, biscuits, pastries, snack foods (e.g. potato crisps, prawn crackers) and changing to skimmed milk and non-fat dairy products.
- **Limit your intake of sugar and sweet foods**, e.g. sweet drinks, sweets, sweet desserts. Have plain water when thirsty, and have fresh fruit after a meal instead of dessert.
- **Increase your fiber intake** to help reduce hunger, e.g. change to wholemeal or multigrain bread instead of white bread, have two servings of

vegetables for lunch and dinner so you will feel less hungry after meals, and choose low fat high-fiber snacks in-between meals when hungry (e.g. boiled chickpeas, fresh fruit, red bean soup, oats, steamed corn).

- **Increase your fluid intake**. Drink at least eight glasses of fluid (including two glasses of skimmed milk) a day. Drinking a glass of water or a bowl of non-cream soup before meals also helps to fill you up, and take the edge off your appetite.

Remember, you should not go on a diet to lose weight when you are pregnant. Instead, focus on eating healthily to control your rate of weight gain so that both you and baby will have optimal nutrition.

FREQUENTLY ASKED QUESTIONS

1. Is it safe to fast during pregnancy?
There are certain concerns with regards to fasting in pregnancy. You may experience hypoglycaemia (low sugar level) with fainting spells as well as giddiness. Also, when fasting is prolonged, the health and growth of the developing baby may be affected. Thus, discuss with your doctor first if you are considering to fast for period or religious reasons during your pregnancy.

2. Can I eat durians during pregnancy?
Durian contains high calories as well as potassium salt. Thus, do eat in moderation or you can gain excessive weight.

3. I have high cholesterol level during pregnancy. Is this a problem?
Pregnancy causes an increase in the blood cholesterol level. This is a normal adaptive response to pregnancy as an ample supply of cholesterol is necessary to maintain fetal development. This level usually normalizes several months after delivery.

There are **no conclusive studies** that show harmful effects of high cholesterol levels to the mother or the developing baby. However, as a high cholesterol level is a risk factor for heart disease and stroke in the long term, we advise you to look into changing your lifestyle if your cholesterol level remains high **after delivery**. Consider a diet low in cholesterol, consisting of bread, fruits, vegetables and small amounts of lean meat, fish and olive oil. Avoid smoking. See your doctor regularly to check your cholesterol level.

Chapter 26

Traditional Chinese Medicine and Pregnancy

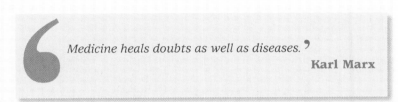

Medicine heals doubts as well as diseases.
Karl Marx

What is Traditional Chinese Medicine (TCM)?

Traditional Chinese Medicine (TCM) is the practice of therapeutic knowledge, which originates from 3000 years of clinical experience through observation and diagnosis. TCM treats a person as an integral biological system and regards that symptoms of diseases do not usually happen alone.

TCM aims to stimulate the body's natural healing potential by treating the root causes and normalizing the body's internal biological balance.

Understanding the Principles of TCM and Women's Health

Typically, a woman will experience menstruation, pregnancy, delivery of new-born as well as breast-feeding at different stages of her life. TCM mainly helps to maintain a good and healthy female reproductive system, as well as study the pathological characteristics of certain reproductive disorders or diseases in an attempt to treat the ailments early to prevent further pathological changes.

"Qi" is a kind of life force or energy that not only refers to the most basic and minute biological substances but also constitutes the human body in order to preserve life.

In TCM, the most important organs that govern the regulation of Qi and Blood are the *liver*, *spleen*, and *kidneys*. The liver is responsible for maintaining a smooth and even flow of Blood and Qi in the body. If the liver malfunctions, it will result in menstrual disorders.

The spleen is the main "factory" which generates Blood and Qi. If the spleen is not functioning, there will be deficiencies in Blood and Qi. This may in turn disrupt the regular menstrual cycles. On the other hand, the kidneys play a big role in excreting the biological waste products and water from the body.

TCM and Habitual Miscarriages

A miscarriage may be triggered by several reasons, which greatly depend on the health status of both the mother and the fetus. Miscarriage may also be related to unhealthy lifestyles such as excessive alcohol intake and smoking. If three consecutive miscarriages occur, this condition is known as **habitual (recurrent) miscarriages**.

In TCM, treatments include replenishing the Qi, nourishing the Blood and strengthening the physiological functions of the spleen. To replenish the body's Qi and nourish the blood reserves, the mother needs to watch her diet and consume proper and nutritious food, such as broccoli, spinach, soya beans, milk and other nutrient-rich food. In addition, she should also have adequate rest with moderate exercise, such as taichi, yoga, frequent slow walks or just simple stretching movements. This ensures the smooth flow of Qi and Blood in the body. There are old grandmother's recipes in TCM such as the red date tea or ginger tea for the day-to-day wellbeing of mothers by constantly and slowly replenishing and nourishing the Qi and Blood in the body.

Red Date Tea (300 ml)
6 pieces of red dates
2 slices of fresh ginger

Bring the red dates to boil for 10 minutes and simmer for another 15 minutes. Add the two slices of fresh ginger while the drink is still hot. Leave to cool to about room temperature before consumption.

Ginger Tea (300 ml)
3–4 slices of fresh ginger
Brown sugar (amount as desired)

Bring the fresh ginger to boil for 5–10 minutes and simmer for another five minutes. Add the brown sugar while the drink is still hot. Leave to cool to about room temperature before consumption.

Chinese Herbs in Pregnancy

The Chinese pay special attention to herbs used for pregnant mothers. TCM

Table 26.1 Classification of Chinese herbs.

Category	Examples
Herbs using animal parts	Centipede（蜈蚣）, Deer musk（麝香）, Freshwater leech（水蛭）
Herbs with natural toxicity	Chuan Wu（川乌）, Cao Wu（草乌）, Fu Zi（附子）
Herbs using natural minerals	Realgar（雄黄）, Gypsum（石膏）, Talcum（滑石）
Herbs with cold properties	Rhubarb（大黄）, Mint（薄荷）, Honeysuckle（金银花）
Herbs with warm properties	Saffron（红花）, Cinnamon bark（肉桂）, Hawthorn berries（山楂）

physicians have formulated many well-known TCM formulations or Chinese prescriptions that are deemed effective to prepare women for different stages in pregnancy.

In order to understand how these prescriptions work, we need to take a closer look at how Chinese herbs interact with each other. According to the basic principles in TCM, every single herb has its own function or group of functions to keep the internal body environment balanced and in harmony. During pregnancy, it is important to keep the Qi (energy flow) and Blood (blood and its related functions) in harmony to ensure a smooth pregnancy.

When a TCM physician puts single herbs or groups of herbs together, he/she produces a prescription. Every TCM herbal prescription is customized for each individual. Therefore, not every formulation is suitable for all. It is prescribed according to each specific set of symptoms of the patients. For example, in TCM, if a patient has fever, herbs with cooling properties will be used.

The herbs in the prescription help restore the internal balance and state of the body and also helps combat some pregnancy-related symptoms, such as nausea and dizziness. Hence, it is important for anxious mothers to understand the principles behind the herbs before they make a decision to take them as medications, nourishments or tonics or as practised in old wives tale. **But a word of caution; if herbs are used inappropriately, side effects such as miscarriages, induced abortions or damages to the fetus may occur.**

The proper combination of herbs is based on their natural functional properties. There are several basic ways Chinese herbs can work together. For example, when herbs with similar properties are used, they enhance or boost the healing power within the entire formulation. Likewise, if herbs of different properties are used, the functions of the herbal couplet may suppress or antagonise the whole formulation.

There are basically two groups of herbs in which pregnant women are advised to keep away from. Table 26.2 shows a list of herbs, which are toxic and uterotonic. These herbs are strictly prohibited for usage during pregnancy.

Table 26.2 Herbs that are **strictly prohibited** for use during pregnancy.

雄黄	Xiong Huang	甘遂	Gan Sui
斑蝥	Ban Mao	大戟	Da Ji
蜈蚣	Wu Gong	芫花	Yuan Hua
马钱子	Ma Qian Zi	牵牛子	Qian Niu Zi
蟾酥	Chan Su	商陆	Shang Lu
川乌	Chuan Wu	麝香	She Xiang
草乌	Cao Wu	水蛭	Shui Zhi
藜芦	Li Lu	虻虫	Meng Chong
胆矾	Dan Fan	三棱	San Leng
瓜蒂	Gua Di	莪术	E Zhu
巴豆	Ba Dou		

Table 26.3 Herbs that are to be **prescribed cautiously** for use during pregnancy.

红花	Hong Hua	大黄	Da Huang
桃仁	Tao Ren	番泻叶	Fan Xie Ye
姜黄	Jiang Huang	芦荟	Lu Hui
牛膝	Niu Xi	天南星	Tian Nan Xing
川芎	Chuan Xiong	芒硝	Mang Xiao
牡丹皮	Mu Dan Pi	附子	Fu Zi
枳实	Zhi Shi	肉桂	Rou Gui
枳壳	Zhi Ke		

(Information of the above herb lists is extracted from the volume of Chinese Materia Medica of the Chinese Pharmacopoeia 《中华人民共和国药典》 published in 2005.)

Table 26.3 shows herbs that should be used with great caution and prescribed only by well-experienced TCM physicians. These herbs are not toxic in nature, but they do have undesirable functions and may cause disruptions to the growing fetus.

Supplements used in Chinese Medicine and their Safety

1. Bird's nest (燕窝 Yan Wo)

Benefits:
   (a) Helps to stimulate appetite and aids in digestion.
   (b) Provides a unique pre-digested form of protein and nutrients that help speed up recovery from chronic illness.

(c) Facilitate normal body functions such as repair of tissues and immunity.

Risks:

In general, no documentation side effects.

2. Chinese Ginseng (中国人参 — Zhong Guo Ren Shen)

Benefits:

(a) Restores strength and energy level after giving birth or severe loss of blood during delivery by improving blood circulation.

(b) Revitalises and aids the recovery process after serious illnesses or major operations by boosting the body's immunity.

(c) Promotes digestion and improves appetite for the mother to produce adequate milk for the newborn.

Risks:

(a) **Do not use when pregnant**.

(b) Not all age groups or medical conditions are suitable to consume Chinese Ginseng.

(c) It should not be taken with high doses of caffeine or other stimulants.

Chinese Ginseng should not be consumed by new mothers who experience hot flushes or skin rashes after delivery.

3. Chinese Angelica Root (当归 Dang Gui)

Benefits:

(a) Commonly used herb in treating many kinds of gynaecological problems such as irregular menstruation, painful menses and infertility.

(b) Efficient in treating anemic conditions.

(c) Commonly used to relieve pain due to blood stagnation, e.g. abdominal pains or traumatic injuries.

(d) This is an important herb for postpartum period, and even during pregnancy as it aims to increase blood production as well as revive a weakened blood circulation.

Risks:

(a) No major side effects with oral administration.

(b) Pregnant women should **consult a licensed TCM physician** before using as it may induce uterine contractions.

(c) May not be wise for women who experience excessive menstrual flow, since this herb promotes better blood circulation.

(d) Used in large doses, Chinese angelica can have adverse effects on blood pressure, heart action and respiration.

4. Royal Jelly (蜂皇浆 Feng Huang Jiang)

Benefits:

    (a) Protects against infections and increases resistance to diseases.

    (b) Accelerates the formation of bone tissue and helps wound healing.

    (c) Moisturizes dry skin and soothes dermatitis.

    (d) Increases endurance and energy levels. It also improves libido.

Risks:

    (a) Allergic reactions (most common) from oral intake of royal jelly can range from very mild (e.g. mild gastrointestinal upset) to more severe reactions, including asthma, anaphylaxis (shock), intestinal bleeding, and even death in people who are extremely allergic to bee products.

    (b) People who are allergic to bee pollen, honey, conifer and poplar trees should not consume oral royal jelly.

    (c) Topical use of royal jelly has been reported to cause skin irritations occasionally.

5. Lingzhi (Ganoderma Lucidum)

Benefits:

    (a) Known as "mushroom of immortality", this fungis is a Qi tonic. It promotes longevity.

    (b) It treats fatigue and enhances immune response.

Risks:

    (a) May cause dizziness and diarrhoea.

    (b) No data on its safety on pregnant women. Use as advised by a TCM physician.

Chapter 27

Safe Medications during Pregnancy and Breastfeeding

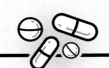

> *Wherever the art of medicine is loved, there is also a love of humanity.*
>
> **Hippocrates**

This chapter contains medications that are commonly used and safe for pregnancy and breastfeeding. This list is not exhaustive and you are advised to consult your doctor before taking medication.

For Common Cold

Medication	Dose	Comments
Chlorpheniramine	4 mg thrice a day	For runny nose Can cause drowsiness
Paracetamol	1 g 6 hourly	For fever, headaches and body aches/pain

For Cough

Dry cough

Medication	Dose	Comments
Dextromethorphan	10 ml thrice a day	Recommended for pregnant and diabetic individuals as it does not contain alcohol
Promethazine/Codeine (Procodin)	10 ml thrice a day	

Productive cough

Medication	Dose	Comments
Diphenhydramine (MBE)	10 ml thrice a day	
Pholcodine/Bromhexine (Durotuss Expectorant)	10 ml thrice a day	Mucolytic agent which does not contain lactose, gluten, color, sugar or alcohol.

Mucolytic (to dissolve thick mucus)

Medication	Dose	Comments
Acetylcysteine (Fluimucil)	600 mg once a day	
Bromhexine	8 mg thrice a day	

Sore throat

Medication	Dose	Comments
Lozenges	1 tablet thrice a day	

For Heartburn and Gastric Pain

Medication	Dose	Comments
Antacids (Examples: MMT, Mylanta, Gelusil, Gaviscon)	Follow instructions on product label	Helps relief bloating and gastric discomfort Take when necessary
Famotidine	20 mg twice a day	
Ranitidine	150 mg twice a day	

For Pregnancy Supplementation

Medication	Dose	Comments
Ascorbic Acid (Vitamin C)	100–200 mg thrice a day	To increase absorption of iron
Caltrate 600	1 to 2 tablets once a day	Each tablet contains 1500 mg calcium carbonate equivalent to 600 mg elemental calcium. Contains no sugar, no salt, no lactose and no preservatives

For Pregnancy Supplementation (con't)

Medication	Dose	Comments
DHA (For example: Natal Care Plus, Neurogain)	Natal Care Plus: 1 to 2 capsules (100 to 200 mg) once a day Neurogain: 1 capsule (250 mg) once a day	Docosahexaenoic acid (DHA) is an omega-3 fatty acid, which is required for baby's normal brain and eye development. The recommended daily intake of DHA during pregnancy is 300 mg daily.
Ferrous Fumarate	200 mg twice a day	Iron supplementation for patients with iron deficiency anemia; contains iron (II) salts
Ferrum Hausmann Syrup	1 ml twice a day	Iron supplementation for patients with iron deficiency anemia; contains iron (III) polymaltose complex with slow release
Floron	1 tablet once a day	Each tablet contains iron hydroxide polymaltose complex and sorbitol which softens stools and causes less constipation
Folic acid	5 mg once a day (or at least 800 micrograms a day)	For peri-conception and first trimester to reduce the risk of neural tube defects (brain and spinal cord abnormalities)
Obimin	1 tablet once a day	Antenatal vitamin supplementation Each tablet contains Vitamin A 3,000 USP units, Vitamin D 400 USP units, Vitamin C 100 mg, Vitamin B1 10 mg, Vitamin B2 2.5 mg, Vitamin B6 15 mg, Vitamin B12 4 mcg, Niacinamide 20 mg, Calcium Panthothenate 7.5 mg, Folic Acid 1 mg, Ferrous Fumarate 90 mg, Calcium Lactate 250 mg, Copper 100 mcg, Iodine 100 mcg
Sangobion	1 tablet once a day	Each capsule contains copper sulfate 200 mcg, ferrous gluconate 250 mg, folic acid 1 mg, manganese sulfate 200 mcg, sorbitol 25 mg, vitamin B12 7.5 mcg, vitamin C 50 mg
Vitacal 250	1 tablet once a day	Each tablet contains 625 mg oyster shell granules (250 mg elemental calcium)

For Threatened Miscarriage (vaginal bleeding in early pregnancy)

Medication	Dose	Comments
Dydrogesterone (Duphaston)	10 mg twice a day	Till 12 weeks of pregnancy
Micronized progesterone (Utrogestan)	100 mg twice a day	
Proluton (Hydroxyprogesterone Caproate)	250 mg once a week	Intramuscular injection after 12 weeks of pregnancy

Anti-Emetics for Nausea and Vomiting

Medication	Dose	Comments
Metoclopramide (Maxolon)	10 mg thrice a day	Intramuscular or intravenous injection Possible **side-effects**: restlessness, drowsiness and fatigue
Promethazine Theoclate (Avomine)	25 mg thrice a day	Possible **side-effects**: drowsiness and fatigue
Pyridoxine	50 mg once a day	Vitamin B6 helps alleviate hyperemesis gravidarum (severe vomiting in pregnancy)

For Constipation

Medication	Dose	Comments
Bisacodyl (Dulcolax) suppository	1 suppository at night	Stimulates gut movements and softens the stools Immediate relief in 15 to 60 minutes
Fleet Enema	Use as diected by your doctor	
Fybogel	1 sachet once a day	Bulk laxative
Lactulose	10 ml twice a day	Stool softener
Liquid Paraffin (Agarol)	10 ml twice a day	Stool softener

Piles during Pregnancy

Medication	Dose	Comments
Bismuth Subgallate (Anusol)	Once a day	Cream/ointment/suppository Reduces pain and inflammation of piles
Diosmin/Hesperidin (Daflon)	2 tabs (500 mg) twice a day	Oral tablet Reduces bleeding and pain of piles
Proctosedyl	Once a day	Ointment/suppository Reduces pain and inflammation of piles Apply sparingly

For Diarrhoea

Medication	Dose	Comments
Charcoal	2 tablets (500 mg) twice a day	Absorbs toxins
Kaolin	10 ml twice a day	Absorbs toxins
Lacteol Forte	1 sachet thrice a day	Contains *Lactobacillus acidophilus* Reduces duration of diarrhoea
Smecta	1 sachet thrice a day	Coats the gut wall for a protective effect

For Lactation Suppression (to stop breast milk flow after delivery)

Medication	Dose	Comments
Cabergoline (Dostinex)	½ tablet twice a day for 2 days	If breastfeeding is initiated
Cabergoline (Dostinex)	2 tablets (single dose)	If breastfeeding is not initiated

Safe Oral Antibiotics during Pregnancy

Medication	Dose	Comments
Amoxycillin	500 mg thrice a day	For urinary tract infection, respiratory tract infection and Group B Streptococcus vaginal infection
Cephalexin	500 mg thrice a day	For urinary tract infection
Erythromycin ethylsuccinate	800 mg twice a day	For those with penicillin allergy

Oral Antibiotics NOT RECOMMENDED in Pregnancy

Medication	Comments
Aminoglycosides (e.g. gentamicin, streptomycin)	To be used with **caution in the second and third trimesters** as they may pose a risk of auditory toxicity (hearing problems) in the developing fetus
Chloramphenicol	Avoid when pregnancy nears term as the infant may not be able to adequately metabolize chloramphenicol. This can result in cardiovascular collapse of baby with high mortality (Grey Baby syndrome)
Quinolones (e.g. Ciprofloxacin)	Avoid in entire pregnancy as it may affect cartilage formation of the fetus
Sulfonamides	**Avoid in the third trimester** as it may cause high bilirubin levels in the baby, resulting in kernicterus (severe jaundice)
Tetracyclines	Avoid in entire pregnancy as it may result in the discoloration of teeth and retard skeletal bone formation of the fetu

For Vaginal Candidiasis (yeast infection) in Pregnancy

Medication	Dose	Comments
Butoconazole (Gynofort) vaginal cream	One time application	Contains butoconazole cream 2%
Clotrimazole pessary	1 pessary once a night for 6 days	Each pessary contains 200 mg clotrimazole
Isconazole (Gynotravogen) pessary	1 pessary once a night for 1 day	Each pessary contains 600 mg isoconazole nitrate
Metronidazole/Nystatin (Flagystatin) pessary	1 pessary once a night for 7 days	Each pessary contains 500 mg metronidazole and 100 000 units nystatin Useful in treating bacterial vaginosis (vaginal infection) as well
Nystatin pessary	1 pessary once a night for 7 days	Each pessary contains 100 000 units nystatin
Tioconazole (Gynotrosyd) pessary	1 pessary once a night for 3 days	Each pessary contains 100 mg tioconazole

For Rash/Itch

Medication	Dose	Comments
Betamethasone valerate (Betnovate) cream	Twice or thrice a day	Topical use Apply thinly
Calamine lotion	To apply when necessary	Topical use
Chlorpheniramine	4 mg three times a day	Can cause drowsiness
Hydrocortisone cream 1%	Twice or thrice a day	Topical use Apply thinly
Isoconazole/Diflucortolone valerate (Travocort) cream	Twice a day	Broad-spectrum anti-fungal with a steroid additive
Miconazole (Daktarin) cream	Twice a day	Anti-fungal cream
Miconazole/Hydrocortisone (Daktacort) cream	Once or twice a day	Broad-spectrum anti-fungal with a steroid additive
Neoderm cream	Contains neomycin and hydrocortisone	Corticosteroid cream with anti-infective agents

Medications for Allergic Rhinitis or Stuffy Nose

Medication	Dose	Comments
Decongestant nasal drops (For example, Afrin, Sinex and Iliadin) **Sudafed is an oral preparation. Oral decongestants are to be avoided during pregnancy**	As directed by the doctor	Some may contain agents which restrict the blood vessels. This may which causes high blood pressure in mother and reduced growth of developing baby **Do not use over-the-counter decongestants.** **See your doctor for advice**
Intranasal steroids (e.g. mometasone, fluticasone)	One spray in each nostril once or twice a day	Contains steroids Use cautiously in pregnancy upon your doctor's advice

Medications for Asthma

Medication	Dose	Comments
Salbutamol inhaler	According to doctor's instructions	To be used only when required for quick-relief of asthma symptoms
Steroidal inhalers (e.g. budesonide, beclomethasone, fluticasone)	According to doctor's instructions	To be used daily for prevention of asthma symptoms. Asthma which is not controlled may cause complications for mother and baby

Table 27.1 FDA classification on safety of medicines used in pregnancy.

FDA Category	Comments
A	Human studies did not show a risk to the developing fetus in pregnancy
B	Animal studies did not show a risk to the developing fetus in pregnancy but there are no studies done in pregnant women
C	Animal studies did show harmful effects on the developing fetus in pregnancy but there are no studies done in pregnant women. Medicine ***should be given*** if the potential benefits justifies the potential risks to the fetus
D	Human studies did show harmful effects on the developing fetus but the benefits from use in pregnant women may be acceptable despite the risk (Examples: the medicine is used in a life-threatening or serious illness)
X	Both human and animal studies show serious harmful effects on the developing fetus. The medicine is ***strictly prohibited*** in pregnancy **(Examples: Chemotherapy drugs and oral isotretinoin.)**

FDA Classification on Safety of Medicines Used in Pregnancy

Since 1975, the U.S. Food and Drug Administration (FDA) assigned pregnancy risk categories to all medicines used in the United States (Table 27.1).

Unfortunately, many medicines have not been adequately researched during pregnancy and due to ethical concerns, will probably not be studied in the future. Thus, please consult your doctor before consuming any medicines in pregnancy.

FREQUENTLY ASKED QUESTIONS

1. **Is taking Evening Primrose Oil (EPO) safe during pregnancy?**
   EPO is a plant extract and commonly used as a dietary supplement. EPO contains linoleic acid, an essential fatty acid. It also contains gamma-linolenic acid, which is important for the production of prostaglandins by the body. Although there are some reports that suggest that EPO might affect the opening of the cervix (neck of womb), there is **insufficient research** *to conclude* if EPO is safe or harmful in pregnancy or even breastfeeding.

2. **Is drinking aloe vera tea safe during pregnancy?**
   Most herbalists would recommend that aloe **not be used in pregnancy** as it may stimulate womb (uterine) contractions. *Remember not to use any herbs* during pregnancy without the approval of your doctor.

3. **Is taking diazepam (sleeping pill) recommended during pregnancy?**
   The information regarding the safety of diazepam is *controversial*. However, several studies have linked the use of diazepam during pregnancy to a small increase in the risk of major malformations (heart and stomach) and cleft palate. Heavy use of diazepam throughout pregnancy has been associated with multiple problems, including dysmorphic features, growth retardation, craniofacial defects, and neonatal withdrawal symptoms. Thus, we **do not recommend its use in pregnancy**.

4. **Is oral or topical tretinoin (Retin-A) safe in pregnancy?**
   Tretinoin (derived from Vitamin A) is given orally or topically to treat acne. Oral tretinoin is **strictly banned in pregnancy** as it causes **multiple malformations** in the developing baby. These include cleft palate, heart and eye anomalies. It can also cause spontaneous miscarriage.

Many children born to mothers who have been treated with tretinoin during pregnancy have reduced IQ and mental impairment.

We also advise to avoid topical Retin-A in pregnancy due to possible skin absorption of the chemical. Instead, **topical erythromycin (an antibiotic) and topical benzoyl peroxide** may be safely used to treat acne.

5. Are over-the-counter (OTC) slimming pills safe in pregnancy?

Many OTC slimming pills contain a combination of herbal products such as Garcinia and Chitosan. The safety profile of slimming pills are *not established* in pregnancy and thus, these slimming pills should be avoided once you are pregnant. Besides, we do not recommend losing weight during pregnancy as the growth of your developing baby may be affected.

6. Is consuming glucosamine safe in pregnancy?

Glucosamine is an endogenous aminomonosaccharide used for the treatment of joint pain (osteoarthritis). There is **insufficient evidence** addressing its safety profile in pregnancy. No adverse outcomes or congenital malformations were reported in pregnant women who had taken glucosamine during pregnancy.

7. Can I use mosquito repellants containing DEET when I am pregnant?

DEET (N,N-ethyl-m-toluamide) is very effective in preventing mosquito bites. This will help protect against mosquito-borne diseases such as malaria and dengue fever. Less than 10% of DEET gets absorbed through the skin. Moreover, animal studies do not show that DEET harms the fetus. The lowest concentration of DEET may be applied onto clothing during pregnancy when protection against insect bites is needed.

8. Are anti-oxidants recommended during pregnancy?

There are some studies, that **recommend antioxidants like vitamin C and E in reducing the risk of pre-eclampsia** (high blood pressure) during pregnancy. In one study, women with pre-eclampsia had significantly lower levels of Vitamin C. In severe pre-eclampsia, vitamin E is also significantly lower; thus, increasing antioxidants during pregnancy may help. Ask your doctor before using these products.

9. Is metronidazole (flagyl) antibiotic considered safe during pregnancy?

FDA has classified Flagyl as a category B drug. Its effect on an unborn child has not been studied extensively. Flagyl should only be used during pregnancy if clearly needed.

10. What pain-killers are safe during pregnancy?

Taking pain-killers like paracetamol is safe during pregnancy as it has no harmful effects on the fetus. Avoid ibuprofen or mefenamic acid which are NSAIDs (non-steroidal anti-inflammatory drugs). This class of drugs is not safe during pregnancy, especially during the last three months. They may affect the baby's circulation, kidney function, or delay the onset of labor. However, there is no evidence that these drugs cause congenital abnormalities.

Chapter 28

Skin Care during Pregnancy

> *Think of stretch marks as pregnancy service stripes.*
> **Joyce Armor**

D uring your pregnancy, many changes can occur on the skin. These changes are related to the surge of female hormones (estrogen and progesterone) to the skin pigments, blood vessels, glands and your immune system. These changes can be physiological or present as skin disorders. The following are seen during pregnancy and improve after delivery.

Pigmentation

You will notice that the color of the nipples, genitalia skin and the center of your tummy darken. Pre-existing freckles and "moles" darken. A dark blemish can appear on your cheeks, forehead, nose and chin called **melasma ("pregnancy mask")** (Figure 28.1). Here, the melanin deposits are increased in the superficial and middle of the skin. Fortunately, the pigment resolves after delivery.

Many women normally have a faint white line (called linea alba) running from their navel to the center of the pubic bone. In the second trimester, this linea alba may darken to be visible. This line is now called **linea nigra**. In some women the line extends upward from the navel as well. The linea nigra is darker in darker skinned women and usually lightens several months after delivery.

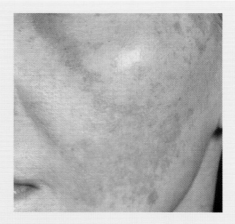

Figure 28.1 Pregnancy mask.

There is another condition with localized pigmentation on the armpits and groins called **acanthosis nigricans** whereby the skin is thickened and dark.

Stretch Marks

The stretching and distension of the tummy causes the skin to split. These split lines are called **striae gravidarum** (Figure 28.2). These are purplish wavy lines, which appear on the tummy, breasts, thighs and groin. After delivery, they become paler in color but the striae remain as permanent scars.

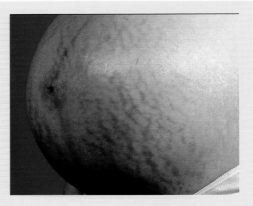

Figure 28.2 Stretch marks.

Blood Vessel Changes

Changes related to blood vessels appear as redness of the palms known as **palmar erythema**; venous varicosities of the legs, vascular lumps on the gums, and "**spider nevi**" or proliferation of blood vessels on the face and chest.

The increased volume of blood also causes the cheeks to take on an attractive blush because of the many blood vessels just below the skin's surface. On top of this redness, the increased secretions of the oil glands give the skin a waxy sheen. Many see this as the "**pregnancy glow**". An increase in the varicose veins may occur in the vulva and vagina at the end of second or third trimester. This may cause a sensation of "heaviness" in the groin.

Hair and Nail Changes

Hair seems to be increased on your scalp with a greater volume. This is because the increased estrogen supports a longer life cycle of your hair. Unfortunately, the increased hair is shed after delivery, and most women are quite upset by the hair lost, and are seen as clumps on the basin as they shampoo their hair. The loss can last three to six months. The hair can increase on your face, back and legs.

Your nails can become brittle and split at the ends.

Acne during Pregnancy

Most women sweat more as their sweat glands become more active. Especially in the third trimester, the oil glands become active and you can develop pimples or acne.

Skin Rash during Pregnancy

The skin becomes very itchy and this is distressing (Figure 28.3). It is due to the impaired transport of bile to the liver and the bile circulates in you body.

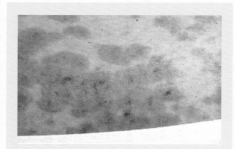

Figure 28.3 Rash during pregnancy.

Some skin diseases get worse during pregnancy. These are eczema, psoriasis, acne, and lupus erythematosus and candidia (fungal) infection of the vagina.

Tips on Skin Care during Pregnancy

- Use a **broad spectrum** sun block on your face each day, to prevent the pigment from further darkening. Avoid the hot sun.
- While mild soap is recommended during pregnancy, **moisturizing soaps** are better. Do not use bubble baths or scrub your skin daily.
- A moisturizer with a **sun block** is helpful. The spf factor or sun protective factor needs to be at least 15 to 20.
- The tummy needs an enriching physiological moisturizer and be supported with special maternity panties. Most women continue to wear their normal panties but these don't support the distending skin. The splits would be less, if these special maternity panties were worn. You need to exercise to keep the abdomen muscles strong. Exercise also reduces stress incontinence. This is a condition where urine leaks out when you cough or sneeze hard. Seaweed wraps and massages are not proven to help.
- Keep your body clean, as you will feel sweaty and hot but limit baths to once a day only. Keep your hair clean with a daily mild shampoo.
- See your doctor if you have bad eczema, as you may need steroid creams but a low potency will have to be prescribed as steroids may thin your skin, if applied in excess.
- Ensure you take vitamins and calcium. Some types of psoriasis get worse with low calcium in your body.
- **Bad acne** can be treated with antibiotic lotions, for example, **erythromycin or clindamycin lotions**. **Do not use tretinoin (Retin-A) cream during pregnancy**, as it is known to cause multiple malformations in the baby.

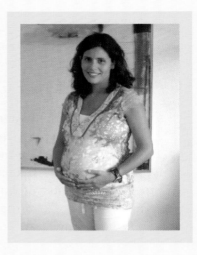

- Reduce intake of foods with a lot of yeast if you have fungal genital infection, like pau, wheat noodles or cakes.
- Have adequate sleep. Adequate exercise helps the skin to glow. **Cosmetics are kept to the basics like sun block, moisturizer, mild cleansers**.
- Above all, be happy and do not overeat as for two. The excess fat gained can be difficult to get rid off later.
- Moisturizers help to decrease the itch. A **physiological moisturizer** like Physiogel cream or Nivea cream is useful. Try not to use paraffin on the skin, as this can clog the skin pores. Chlorpheniramine tablets can be taken to relieve the itch.

Tips on Skin Care after Delivery

As there are at least three months of postpartum care for the working mother and a much longer time for mothers who are not working, you need to get your skin back to normal.

- Exercises may tone up your abdomen and reduce the striae.
- **Low potency vitamin A cream** will help improve the scars in the tummy. As you will be tired looking after the child, try to get enough sleep and do allow others to help with looking after the child. You need to be well rested and happy.
- The breasts may be sore from the baby sucking too vigorously on the nipple: Allow the child to suck properly on the areolar area as well. Clean the nipple area and moisturize them.
- Continue to use a **sunblock** and a **lightening cream called hydroquinone cream** to clear the melasma.
- Continue to use **moisturizers** on your body daily, especially after the bath.
- For excessive hair loss, you can use **minoxidil spray** on your scalp.
- Any remaining acne, you can use **topical antibiotics, oxy cream** and a **vitamin A cream** in the evening.
- Should you or your baby develop any skin rashes, consult a doctor.
- Use a **silicone gel sheet** or **silicone cream** on your cesarean section wound to reduce the chance of keloid formation (overgrowth of fibrous tissue at cesarean wound).

Safety of Makeup and Skin/Hair Care Products during Pregnancy

Exposure to certain environmental agents during pregnancy can lead to birth defects, abnormal fetal growth and pregnancy complications. For most skin and hair care products, the evidence of harm during pregnancy is *not established*. Not all products have been studied adequately in pregnancy.

Chemicals from certain skin and hair care products can be absorbed through the skin and into the bloodstream. Thus, if you want to protect your developing baby from unnecessary chemical exposure, especially during the first trimester when critical organ systems are developing, you may want to avoid using these products while you are pregnant.

Products such as shampoos, hair sprays, soaps, lotions and deodorants have not been shown to be harmful during pregnancy. Using these products are generally safe. It is also not known if the chemicals used in artificial nail products are safe for use by anyone, whether you're pregnant or not. Nail removers contain ingredients that are extremely toxic if ingested. Avoid prolonged inhalation of fumes from nail products.

Tattoos during Pregnancy

Body art, which includes piercing, tattoos and permanent make-up, has various health risks. The risks most relevant to pregnancy include the safety of the dyes and the possibility of infections or allergic reactions. Because the skin is punctured for all body art procedures, there is a risk that a local infection could develop at the puncture site. There is also a small risk that blood-borne infections could be transmitted, such as HIV or hepatitis B or C, from improperly disinfected body art tools. With a tattoo or permanent make-up, ink is injected into the second layer of skin. The **safety of this ink is unknown**. Some inks are approved for skin application as cosmetics, but their safety when injected into the skin has not been thoroughly studied.

DID YOU KNOW?

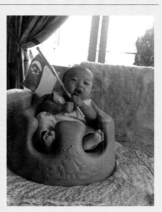

- Your baby is considered full term after **37 weeks** gestation and will put on about 200 grams every week.
- At **40 weeks** gestation, your baby is about 50 cm long and weighs an average of 3000 grams.
- All your baby's organs are functioning and baby is now ready for survival outside the womb.

Chapter 29

Dental Care during Pregnancy

> *Oral health is just as important as getting a regular physical. It's not just about getting a cavity filled, it's about the overall health of the individual.*
>
> **Jennifer Williams**

Starting Right

One cannot over-emphasize the importance of preventive dental care to maintain a healthy set of teeth and gums. Taking charge of your dental health for a healthy pregnancy starts even before you conceive. This minimizes dental uncertainties and enables you to concentrate on your pregnancy. You should visit your dentist for a check up, scaling and polishing of your teeth.

Gum Disease in Pregnancy

Pregnancy increases the risk for developing gingivitis and periodontitis (gum infection) due to the increase in estrogen and progesterone.

Gingivitis (bleeding gums) is an inflammation of the gums, which appear red and swollen. You may find that they bleed easily, especially when you brush your teeth. This is most commonly seen between the second and eighth months of pregnancy (Figure 29.1).

Periodontitis is a more severe form of gingivitis, involving destruction of the supporting bone structure surrounding the teeth. This may result in your teeth becoming shaky. You may even lose the affected teeth if the condition is allowed to deteriorate.

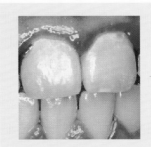

Figure 29.1 Gum disease.

It is important to adopt the correct practice to prevent periodontitis as studies have shown a link between periodontal disease and premature delivery.

Preventing Gum Disease

Adopting good oral hygiene is essential to prevent gum disease. This includes brushing after each meal, flossing at least once a day, and using an anti-plaque mouth rinse.

Visit the dentist regularly at least every six months to check that your gums are healthy and for professional cleaning of your teeth. This should be practised even prior to conception, to ensure healthy gums right from the start of pregnancy.

Caries (Dental Decay)

Being pregnant by itself does not cause dental decay, but the symptoms associated with it may indirectly result in caries. Morning sickness and tiredness in the first trimester can result in dental neglect and poor oral health. This increases one's risk to caries. In addition, food cravings during pregnancy may result in higher or more frequent sugar intake, also increasing the risk of developing caries.

Making the extra effort to practise good oral hygiene (brushing after meals, flossing once a day and using a fluoride mouth rinse) is thus essential to prevent caries.

Amalgam Fillings (Silver Fillings)

During pregnancy

You can be exposed to inorganic mercury from the inhalation of mercury vapor released from amalgam fillings, especially greatest during the placement or removal of the filling.

While it is comforting to know that existing amalgam fillings in the mouth do not pose a risk of mercury toxicity to the fetus during pregnancy, there has been a concern of mercury toxicity during the placement or removal of amalgam fillings in pregnancy. The good news is that there has been no evidence to prove this relationship. Similarly, there is no evidence to confirm that placement or removal of amalgam fillings during pregnancy increases the risk of low birth weight of the baby.

However, as a precautionary measure, you should **avoid any unnecessary procedures involving amalgam**, if possible. You may discuss with your dentist about using an alternative filling material such as tooth-colored resins, which do not contain mercury.

During breastfeeding

Mercury from amalgam fillings can also be transferred into breast milk. However, it has not been determined if the measured amount of mercury in the breast milk is a result of mercury from the amalgam fillings or from dietary exposure, such as the consumption of fish.

While there is **insufficient evidence** to suggest that placement and removal of amalgam fillings whilst breastfeeding can cause mercury toxicity to the baby, it would still be prudent to **avoid such procedures**, if possible, until breastfeeding has stopped.

Radiographs

Dental X-rays are of very low dosage and pose little harm. However, to be cautious, **dental radiographs should only be taken during pregnancy if there is an emergency.**

Some dental infections may spread to other parts of the head and neck region and need to be treated. Any trauma to the teeth may also be considered a dental emergency. In circumstances like these, dental radiographs are indicated.

A **lead apron over the abdomen** can be worn to protect your baby from radiation when dental radiographs are taken, so there should be no cause for worry.

Pregnancy Tumor

The term "pregnancy tumor" sounds and looks intimidating, but is actually less serious than it portrays itself to be. The pregnancy tumor is also known as "pyogenic granuloma" or "pregnancy epulis".

It is a **benign growth at the gum margin** that can become quite large and bleed easily upon trauma (Figure 29.2). This is due to an extreme inflammatory response to local irritation such as plaque and is **most common in the second trimester.** A large pregnancy tumor may be uncomfortable and can cause difficulty in speech and eating.

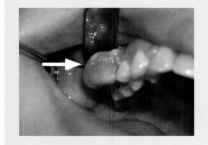

Figure 29.2 Pregnancy tumor (as shown by arrow).

Preventing Pregnancy Tumors

Maintaining good oral hygiene and regularly receiving professional cleaning reduces your risk of a pregnancy tumor developing.

Treatment of Pregnancy Tumors

Pregnancy tumors usually **resolve spontaneously after delivery**. Thus, leave the pregnancy tumor alone if it does not cause you too much inconvenience, but continue to maintain good oral hygiene. However, if it causes discomfort or **affects your speech or eating**, you may wish to seek treatment from your dentist. Pregnancy tumors may be **excised surgically under local anesthesia**. This is a minor procedure and should not be a cause for alarm.

FREQUENTLY ASKED QUESTIONS

1. **Are dental procedures safe during pregnancy?**
   While regular check-ups and cleaning are highly recommended during pregnancy, elective major dental procedures (for example bleaching) should be postponed till after delivery of your baby. If fillings are required, amalgam should be avoided and an alternative filling material be used instead.

   As the first trimester is the most critical period of your baby's development, dental treatment, if necessary, is **best performed in the second trimester** to minimize risk. Discuss your dental needs with your dentist.

   Treatment in the third trimester is often not recommended due to the unfavourable supine position during treatment. This position affects your blood circulation as it slows down blood flow back to the heart. Do inform your dentist if you are not comfortable and adjust the dental chair accordingly.

   In the unique situation where you may be undergoing braces treatment and got pregnant, adjustment of the braces is *safe* throughout pregnancy.

2. **Are braces safe for patients who are undergoing cesarean section?**
   Many patients wearing braces have no problems with surgery and anesthesia. However, do inform the anesthetist if you are undergoing general anesthesia to take special precautions not to dislodge the braces during intubation of the airway.

Chapter 30

Role of the New Father

> The most important thing a father can do for his children is to love their mother. ✎
>
> **Theodore M Hesburgh**

The importance of the support of your partner as a father cannot be understated. As pregnancy and delivery is a shared experience, the "new" father must offer as much moral, emotional and physical support as he possibly can. Indeed, many would be excited about the prospect of being a father.

Keep Up-to-date about Your Pregnancy

While you are coping with the physical demands of the pregnancy, your partner can help immensely by doing the reading and educating you. In this way, your partner will feel involved in the pregnancy.

Being well informed about various aspects of pregnancy, your partner can reassure you about the milder ailments and symptoms such as backache, leg cramps or even Braxton Hicks pains later in the pregnancy.

See Your Obstetrician Together

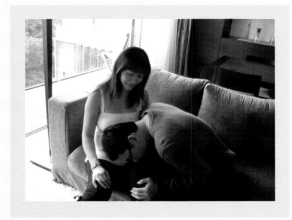

It is a lovely sight to see your partner attending the clinic with you. Encourage him to come along and ask questions about the pregnancy. If your partner has a family history of significant medical problems such

as Down Syndrome or thalassemia, it is useful for him to
communicate this to your doctor. More tests can then be performed to ascertain such risks
in your baby.

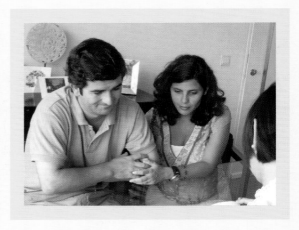

Ask questions and be in-
volved in the decision process
such as deciding on whether
to go ahead with the various
Down Syndrome screening
tests. Knowing the progress of
the pregnancy will enable the
father to understand the physical and emotional demands that you face.

Seeing your baby on the ultrasound scan together will help him feel the
emotional bonding immediately. He will feel just as excited and thrilled as
you.

It will be great if both of you can attend the antenatal preparation classes
together. Getting to know more about the symptoms of pregnancy will help
your partner understand and appreciate what you are going through. He surely
will not mind massaging your calves in the middle of the night when you experience leg cramps. He will also better understand your mood swings, appetite
changes and sudden cravings.

Your Partner's Role during Delivery

Discuss your birth plan together with your obstetrician. Your partner's presence
at delivery is your best emotional support. However, be realistic if your partner
has a fear of blood. (We have had to attend to several fathers who collapsed
at the sight of blood!)

Ask the father to watch when the baby's head is just appearing at the
vaginal opening. And very often, your partner's encouragement is the best
motivation for you at this critical moment.

Most fathers love to cut the umbilical cord for the babies and we often
encourage this. Indeed, this would signify the first responsibility of the new
father. Armed with digital video cameras, most fathers would be the proud
photographer of these precious moments of the newborn.

Birth and delivery is miraculous. Both of you must enjoy this emotional
experience together!

The New Father

Communication and support is absolutely essential especially in the first few days after delivery. Your partner must understand the possible mood swings and postnatal "blues" that many new mothers face in the first week. You will need all the physical and emotional support that he can provide.

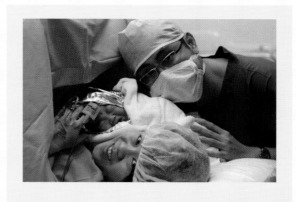

As a new father, he may be caught up with the various new tasks of fatherhood such as changing diapers and helping with feeds. Be open and communicate with him about your needs. You will want to feel loved. Explore the issue of sexual intimacy and contraception as well (see Chapter 51 on "Resuming sexual relations and contraception").

Above all, becoming a new father is an incredible life experience. Savor it!

DID YOU KNOW?

Taking pictures of the precious moments of your baby's milestone developments will help you increase the bonding with your child. Your child will appreciate them when he/she grows up.

One of the authors during his childhood days. Guess who he is?

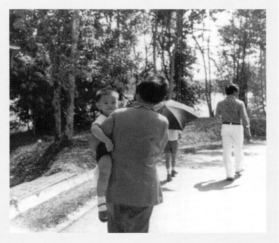

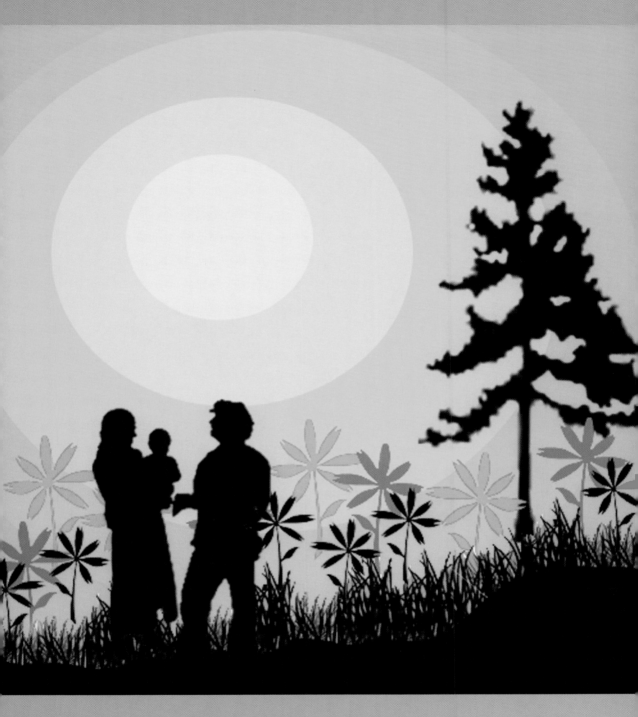

Concerns About Your Delivery

Chapter 31

Birth Plan and Role of a Doula

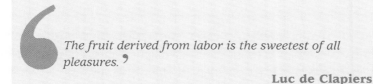

> 'The fruit derived from labor is the sweetest of all pleasures.'
>
> **Luc de Clapiers**

Childbirth is not just about the delivery of a baby. It is also a very special experience for both mum and dad. Many women appreciate having choices in their childbirth and a birth plan is a good way of communicating these choices to your obstetrician. It is best to discuss your birth plan with your obstetrician well ahead of time.

What is a Birth Plan?

A birth plan is not a contract. It is a platform for communication between your partner, care givers and you. It is important that you know what the reasons are and what the implications your alternative choices will have on you and your baby.

Who Should I Involve?

You should indicate your wishes to your obstetrician, midwives and delivery suite staff when you go into labor. Sometimes, it is useful to discuss your options with your obstetrician during the antenatal consultation. Some women will discuss their birth plans with their doctors although birth plans are not common practices here.

What are the Limitations That May Be Faced?

Certain hospitals have various policies such as allowing only one member of your family into the delivery room, or prohibiting the presence of the partner during a cesarean section due to various logistic and infrastructural considerations. Discuss with your obstetrician to find out more about these hospital regulations. This enables you and your doctor to decide on a reasonable consensus between your ideals and the standard care given to you and your baby at delivery.

It is also important to appreciate that the process of childbirth can sometimes be unpredictable and may not necessarily go the way you expect. In these situations, your obstetrician will guide you as to what is medically the best solution for you and your baby.

What are Some of The Issues That can Be Considered?

Not everyone needs or wants a formal and written birth plan. What is important is that you should have a detailed discussion with your doctor in the antenatal period regarding the process of labor, methods of pain relief and any other concerns. This will make the childbirth more meaningful for you and your partner.

Most people have preferences for how things are to be done during the labor and birth.

A birth plan might address some of these issues:

During labor

- Do you prefer to ambulate or do you wish to be confined to a bed?
- Do you prefer an intravenous drip, intravenous access, or none at all?
- Do you prefer to wear your own clothing?
- Do you prefer to be able to have some drinks and small snacks during labor?
- Do you prefer to listen to music?
- Do you prefer to use the birth pool or have a shower? (Only certain hospitals have the earlier option and there are some pros and cons associated with this, so please discuss this in detail with your doctor.)
- Do you prefer pain relief or do you want to avoid them? (see Chapter 37)
- Do you have any preferences for which pain medications you want?
- Would you prefer a certain position in which to give birth — semi-sitting/standing/kneeling?
- Would you prefer an episiotomy? Or, are there certain measures to avoid one? (Refer to Chapter 38 for the advantages of an episiotomy.)
- If you need a cesarean section, do you have any special requests?

After delivery

- Would you like your partner to cut the cord?
- Would you like to claim the placenta?
- Would you like to store the cord blood?
- Would you like to hold onto the baby immediately after giving birth?
- Would you like to breast feed immediately?

It is important to exercise flexibility on your requests, especially if it compromises on the care and safety of your delivery. Please consult your obstetrician as he or she will know what is best for you and your baby.

Role of a Doula

"Doula" in Greek literally means a woman's servant. This refers to a woman trained as a labor companion. There are various roles that a doula may assume prior to your delivery and that depends very much on your own preferences. However, there are also doulas available for antenatal or post-partum care.

The doula will not be able to replace your doctor or midwife in managing your labor. When in labor, she will serve as an additional source of support and accompany you right through the process — providing you with the necessary psychological and emotional care. She would also advice you on relaxation techniques, breathing exercises and labor positions. Even after delivery, she would assist you in your postnatal care and breastfeeding. Good doulas will even involve the father in the plans so that he will not feel left out.

Many studies show that doulas can enhance your birth experience, reduce the need for pain relief in labor and shorten labor. However, it is imperative that the final care of your labor and the mode of delivery are made after consulting your obstetrician.

When choosing a doula, it is important to establish her prior experience, training, the type of services that she provides and her availability at the time of your delivery. It is also advisable to have an interview so that you could discuss your birth plan with her in advance.

Chapter 32

Am I in Labor?

> *Just as a woman's heart knows how and when to pump,*
> *her lungs to inhale,*
> *and her hand to pull back from fire,*
> *So she knows when and how to give birth.*
>
> **Virginia Di Orio**

Many women who have experienced childbirth remain puzzled about this elusive entity known commonly as "labor". There are also many versions of laboring symptoms and signs contributed by friends and relatives. Among those include back pain, tummy pain, bladder pain, bleeding from vagina, bursting of water bag and constipation-like symptoms. No two women may experience the same thing. A woman who had more than one child commonly has different experiences for each of her labor.

Labor is characterized by:

- Painful womb contractions
- Progressive dilatation of the neck of the womb (cervix)
- Possible rupture of the amniotic membranes with leakage of liquor or passing out of a mucous plug or bloody show.

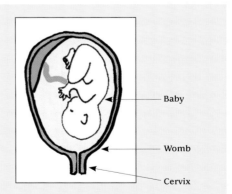

Figure 32.1 Schematic diagram showing the relationship of the baby, womb and cervix.

Painful Uterine Contractions

This is a necessary component of labor. Womb contractions that are associated with increasing pain signal the dilation of the cervix and the possible onset of labor. Contractions that are not associated with pain are probably **"Braxton Hicks"** or commonly known as "practice" contractions or false labor pains. These painless contractions do not cause opening of the cervix.

In the majority of cases, the pain associated with labor is severe; although this may start out as moderate. It is less common that women experience the true labor pains associated with progressive cervical dilation without requesting some form of pain killers. One distinguishing feature of labor pains is that it is episodic. Women describe that the pain/contraction builds up and last for 10–60 seconds, and then subsides spontaneously. This same character of pain returns between 5 minutes and 30 minutes.

Your labor is considered established when the contraction increases in **duration** (e.g. commonly lasting at least 30 seconds) and **frequency** (e.g. occurring every 5–10 minutes). This is associated with opening of the cervix to 3–4 cm.

Progressive Cervical Dilatation

A vaginal assessment is necessary to determine the opening of the cervix. This is usually well tolerated by patients except in patients with **vaginismus**, a condition characterized by the involuntary squeezing of the pelvic muscles upon insertion of the examining fingers. The use of **adequate pain relief such as entonox or epidural** helps greatly in such cases. In addition, staying calm and relaxed in the presence of a supportive partner is also helpful.

In modern obstetrics, the husband/partner of the patient stands by her side to support her during such an assessment. The patient lies on her back and

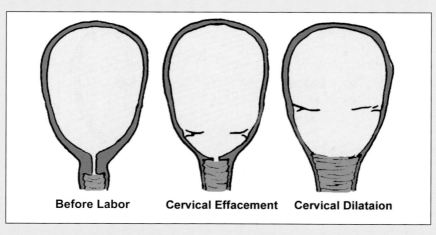

| Before Labor | Cervical Effacement | Cervical Dilataion |

Figure 32.2 Cervical dilata tion at different stages of labor.

relaxes her thighs to either side. Gentle cleansing is done to the exterior. In between contractions, the examiner inserts two digits (that are well lubricated with obstetric cream) gently into the birth canal. Breathing exercises may help in relaxation during this process. If you are allergic to the cream that is commonly used, alternative solutions may be used.

The examiner is able to assess your labor by determining the **opening of the cervix** in centimeters, the *texture* (soft or firm), *position* (front or back), *station* (head is low or high), and *effacement* (thin or thick). Established labor is associated with wider opening, soft texture, front position, thin cervix and low head. There is a need to re-examine you again a few hours later to confirm that your cervix is dilating and that your labor is progressing normally. The cervix is considered fully dilated when the opening is 10 cm.

Additional signs of labor

Rupture of your membranes will present as **"a gush of warm straw-colored fluid"** between your legs. This can be distinguished from urine as it will feel warm and smell sweetish, unlike the strong ammonia smell of urine. If your baby has **passed motion**, the fluid will be yellowish or greenish instead. This leakage tends to be continuous till your baby delivers. Once this happens, you must head for the hospital regardless of the presence of the other symptoms. About 80% of women with ruptured membranes will go into established labor pains within 24 hours of the event. 90% of women will go into established labor within 48 hours.

The **mucous plug** is a gelatinous substance that covers the opening of your womb in pregnancy. Passing out of this plug may herald the onset of labor proper, but it may take hours or days before labor actually starts. Bloody show presents itself as a mucoid discharge that is tinged brownish. Like the mucous plug, it may be a sign that the cervix is dilating and labor is about to begin soon.

There is no time line to deliver the baby after experiencing a show or mucous plug. The pre-requisites of painful uterine contractions associated with progressive cervical dilation must be present for established labor.

Pain in the uterus that is continuous and severe without respite may indicate premature separation of the placenta from the uterus (**abruption placenta**). This is a **serious condition** that requires immediate access to hospital. This condition is also associated with fresh red vaginal bleeding (unlike bloody show) and unrelenting pain.

One reason why labor remains elusive is that the trigger and sustenance is unpredictable.

Some scenarios commonly encountered in the delivery suite

1. A patient describes having painful contractions for about 10–15 seconds that occur every 30 minutes. The pain settles down and she is in no pain after about 4 hours. A vaginal examination showed that the cervix is closed.

   Comment: This is a common scenario seen in maternity hospitals. As the cervix is closed despite the description of painful contractions earlier, the **patient is not in labor**. The contractions were not sufficient to cause opening of the cervix (i.e. no work is done despite the pain). Painful contractions may subside and may not recur even after many days.

2. A patient describes having painful uterine contractions for 30 seconds that lasts every 10 minutes. A vaginal examination showed that the cervix is 2 cm dilated.

   Comment: **This patient is in "early labor"**. The painful contractions had resulted in some "work done" as reflected in the opening of the cervix to 2 cm. However, even at this stage, the contractions may subside resulting in no further natural progress. Some of these patients opt to go home after being monitored during the contraction phase in hospital. Others may opt for induction of labor.

3. A patient describes having painful uterine contractions for 30 seconds that lasts every five minutes and appears to be getting closer. A vaginal examination showed that the cervix is 4 cm dilated.

   Comment: This patient has painful, regular contractions that persist and the cervix is opening. **She is in established labor.**

Premature Labor (i.e. < 37 Completed Weeks of Pregnancy)

Some women experience premature labor pains. The character is similar to normal labor pains. Premature labor is commonly more rapid and may result in the expulsion of the baby soon after labor begins. Hence, many doctors are cautious in evaluating pain in the second and early third trimester to identify premature labor pains and to arrest it early. Women who experience possible labor pains before 36 weeks gestation should consult their obstetrician promptly.

What if I Cannot Get to the Hospital on Time?

Most of the time, our patients are able to seek medical attention before the baby delivers. Occasionally, we still do have mothers who deliver before they can reach the hospital. Such an occurrence is more common in those who have delivered before and labor pains may be mistaken for insignificant abdominal cramps. It is also more common in those with a history of rapid labor or precipitous labor, whereby the baby delivers within a few hours of the onset of labor. Should this ever happen to you, the following is a suggested guide on what should be done (see Figure 32.4):

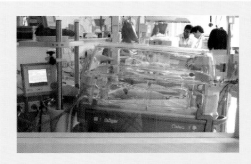

Figure 32.3 Neonatal Intensive Care Unit with premature babies in incubators.

- **Remain calm at all times**. The last thing you and your partner should do is to panic.

- **Call for help**. This includes dialing for the ambulance (995) and alerting your neighbors or someone to come and assist you.

- **Prepare for your delivery**:
  a. Lie down on a bed or sofa while awaiting medical help.
  b. Spread some clean towels under yourself.
  c. If possible, your partner should wash his hands and your vaginal area.
  d. Avoid pushing as this may expedite the delivery. In times like this, deep breathing may help distract you.

- **Delivering your baby**:
  a. Should you or your partner start to see the baby's head, then you should help by pushing each time you feel the urge to bear down.
  b. Let the head emerge on its own. Never attempt to pull it out and should there be a loop of umbilical cord around the neck, you or your partner should gently hook it over the baby's head.
  c. Once the head is delivered, hold it gently with two hands and press it downwards so that the anterior shoulder can be delivered under your pelvic bones.
  d. Once the anterior shoulder is delivered, you may gently lift the head so that the posterior shoulder can be freed.

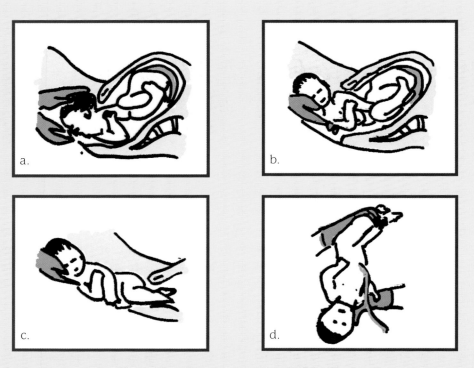

Figure 32.4 Steps in normal vaginal delivery.

- **After your delivery:**
  a. Keep the baby warm by wrapping him/her in a clean towel, before placing it on your abdomen.
  b. Do not attempt to cut or pull onto the umbilical cord.
  c. Should the placenta deliver spontaneously, manually rub the uterus by placing your hands onto the lower part of your abdomen. This will promote the contraction of your womb and reduces the blood loss.
  d. Make yourself comfortable while help is on its way.

Chapter 33

What to Pack and What to Expect in the Delivery Suite?

> *Hope is a desire with an expectation of accomplishment.*
>
> **Anonymous**

What Do I Need before Coming to the Hospital?

A common question, especially for first time parents, is "What do I need to pack for the hospital?" Do not be daunted by the huge size of this suggested list — you do not have to bring all the things that are listed here. The idea here is to have a comprehensive list that you can pick and choose from. This enables you to customize your own list of the things so that you can feel comfortable at the end of the day.

Here are some suggestions:

1. **For Mom:**

   Toiletries
   - Lotion
   - Toothbrush and toothpaste
   - Hairbrush/comb
   - Shampoo/soap
   - Towel/facecloth

   Clothing
   (You will be wearing a hospital gown during your delivery.)
   - Two loose fitting nighties — preferably the breastfeeding kind (if you are not keen to use the hospital gown which are made for breastfeeding)
   - A pair of slippers

- Few pairs of underwear
- Socks
- Nursing bra
- Clothing to wear upon discharge from the hospital

Birth plan — if you do have one (see Chapter 31).

2. For Dad:

- Some reading material when your spouse is sleeping or resting
- Toiletries
- Change of clothes
- Sweater

3. For Baby:

- One baby outfit upon discharge
- Receiving blanket
- One pair of socks or booties
- One pair of mittens
- Cap

After Delivery:

- Name list of people to call once baby arrives. You will inevitable forget to call someone.
- Digital camera/camcorder — to capture all those precious moments.

Do Not Bring:

- Valuables
- Jewelry
- Laptop computer

What Happens When I Arrive at the Delivery Suite?

You will be attended to by the midwife and the doctor-on-duty, who will assess whether you are in labor or not at the triage area situated at the entrance of the de-

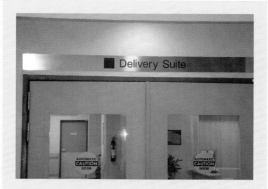

Figure 33.1 Delivery Suite at KK Hospital.

livery suite. Based on your condition, you will be either admitted to the delivery suite, antenatal ward, or advised to return home with a follow up appointment to see your obstetrician.

What Do I Expect in the Delivery Suite?

Once admitted, you will be directed into one of the rooms by one of the staff. Monitoring is done to follow the course of labor (whether you are progressing normally) and to find out the status of the fetus during labor.

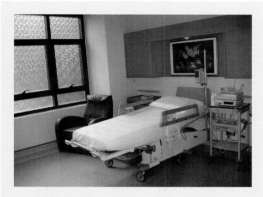

Figure 33.2 A room in the delivery suite.

Your Doctor/Nurse will be Monitoring the Following in the Delivery Suite:

- Your **vital parameters** such as general condition, pulse rate, blood pressure and temperature on a 4-hourly basis.

- A **cardiotocograph** will probably be used, whereby a strap will be gently placed around your abdomen to allow us to monitor the following:
  o The frequency and intensity of your uterine contractions — medication may be needed to help increase the contractions so that labor can progress normally.
  o The continuous monitoring of your baby's heart rate — this helps us to detect any abnormal patterns of the baby's heart rate so that appropriate interventions may be administered.

  This may be performed at a half-hourly interval or for a continuous period till your baby is delivered. A continual beeping sound will be emitted during the monitoring process, so do not be alarmed as the volume can be adjusted accordingly.
  The use of this monitor is safe for you and your baby.

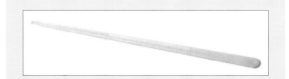

Figure 33.3 Amniohook used to rupture the membranes.

- **Periodic internal vaginal examination**: Your doctor or nurse may do an internal examination periodically (usually at 4 hourly intervals) or as the situation requires. An internal examination is performed to assess the progress of labor and 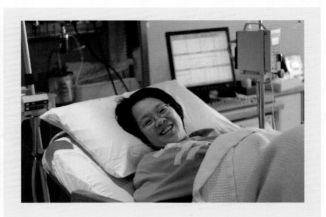 the color of the amniotic fluid, which may be a reflection of your baby's well being during the course of labor. If your bag of waters is not yet ruptured, the doctor may do so using an **amniohook** when your cervix is dilated to about 3 cm. This procedure should be painless if you are well relaxed. You may feel some warm fluid trickling down your vulva and buttocks.
- An intravenous (IV) line may be inserted to administer IV fluids or other medications. This is especially important if you are kept nil-by-mouth or fasted as this prevents dehydration.

Common Medications Used during Labor

- **Analgesics** for pain relief to prevent or decrease labor pains (see Chapter 37).
- **Oxytocics** to increase the effectiveness of uterine contractions so that the labor can progress normally. After your delivery, these medications will be used to reduce the amount of blood loss by promoting effective womb contractions.
- **Antibiotics** may be given intravenously to reduce the chance of infections under certain circumstances, such as in those with Group B streptococcus infections or prolonged rupture of membranes or maternal pyrexia/fever.
- A **fleet enema** may be given to you to help empty your bowels before your delivery.
- **Medicines** that may have been prescribed for you during your pregnancy will be continued to be served during your labor such as antiepileptic or thyroid medications.

Breastfeeding After Your Delivery

Many women prefer to breastfeed because it is natural and helps to provide the baby with the necessary antibodies to protect him/her from illness and disease. Immediately after the delivery, your baby will be handed to you for the early initiation of breastfeeding. This will facilitate subsequent successful breastfeeding, and promote close bonding between mother and baby (see Chapter 45).

FREQUENTLY ASKED QUESTIONS

1. What documents should I bring along?
In addition to the above-mentioned items, you should bring along your outpatient appointment booklet, identity cards of both mum and dad, marriage certificate and admission form.

2. What happens when I arrive at the delivery suite?
You will be attended to by the midwife and the doctor-on-duty, who will assess whether you are in labor or not. Based on your condition, you will be either admitted to the delivery suite, antenatal ward, or advised to return home with a follow up appointment to see your obstetrician.

3. What can I do to help myself?
- As far as your labor pains are concerned, in addition to the analgesia, you may try a variety of self-help methods like relaxation, deep breathing, etc.
- Keep yourself adequately hydrated — take ice chips to counter your thirst.
- A frequent mouth wash such as a periodic gargle can help you feel fresh and good.
- Pass urine frequently as a full bladder may impede labor. If you are unable to void, you may require a catheterization to empty your bladder.
- Using a damp cloth to wipe your face and body can help you feel refreshed.
- Having your spouse by your side throughout the labor can provide you with great physical and moral support. Your partner can massage your back, distract you and provide comfort and reassurance. This can be a great help in calming you down and helping you enjoy your labor.

- During the first stage of labor, remember not to push nor strain. Always make a conscious effort and tell yourself to relax in between your contractions. Pushing during this stage will not help in your progress in anyway.
- Your first stage will last for an average of 8–12 hours from onset of labor. So remember that you will not deliver as soon as you are in the hospital (see Chapter 35).

Chapter 34

Induction of Labor (IOL)

> Only with trust, faith, and support can the woman allow the birth experience to enlighten and empower her.
>
> **Claudia Lowe**

What Causes Labor?

The exact mechanisms causing labor in pregnant mothers are uncertain. However, it is very likely that there is a series of events involving various hormones, genes and other substances within your body, resulting in the dual process of contractions in the womb and opening of the neck of the womb (cervix). It is also believed that this is initiated by the baby and the placenta.

What is Induction of Labor (IOL)?

You may have heard this term many times, but do you know what it means? Induction of labor (IOL) is any medical intervention performed that stimulates the onset of labor pains (i.e. to establish labor), aiming to result in the delivery of the baby vaginally (see Chapter 35).

Do I Really Need to Undergo IOL?

A variety of medical conditions may arise during the course of your pregnancy that may put you or your baby's well being at risk. This may necessitate your doctor offering you an early delivery of your baby. In certain instances where you or your baby is assessed to be unable to tolerate the stress of labor, a *cesarean section* may be suggested to expedite your delivery instead. Only if time permits and there is no immediate danger to you or your baby, an IOL can then be offered.

What are the Medical Reasons that May Necessitate IOL?

These can be broadly categorized into conditions that can put either you or your baby at risk should the pregnancy be allowed to progress. Under such a circumstance, your doctor would have investigated you thoroughly and assessed that it would be safer for either mother or baby that the delivery occurs before your due date or in rarer cases, even before maturity is reached.

- **Pre-eclampsia (PE)** is a serious medical disorder caused by pregnancy. PE may affect many organs but commonly manifests as high blood pressure, leaking of protein in the mother's urine and generalized swelling in the mother (see Chapter 21). Delivery of the baby will treat PE and reduce the risk of harm. Hence IOL is commonly performed before the mother reaches the severe stage of PE.
- **Diabetic mothers** are commonly induced before their estimated delivery date. Babies of diabetic mothers are commonly larger and early delivery makes it less challenging. Babies of diabetic mothers are also at increased risk of stillbirth, if not delivered by the due date (especially if the sugar control is poor).
- **Intrauterine growth restriction (IUGR)** means that the baby is not growing to his/her full potential (see Chapter 21). It is preferable to deliver the baby and provide nutrition externally.
- **Intrahepatic cholestasis of pregnancy (ICP)** is a condition which presents with generalized skin itch in the mother. There is also evidence of liver dysfunction. ICP is associated with stillbirth and IOL at 37–38 weeks is often recommended to prevent this.
- Women with a personal history of **precipitous labor** (i.e. very rapid delivery) are commonly offered IOL after 37 weeks of gestation for practical reasons. In subsequent labor, their risk of rapid delivery remains high and the time from onset of pain to expulsion of baby may be less than 60 minutes. Hence, IOL offers certainty of professional assistance.
- **Post-date** is a condition whereby your pregnancy goes past the expected due date. An IOL may then be offered. Studies have indicated that an IOL under these circumstances would reduce the incidence of stillbirth and the need to perform a cesarean section for fetal distress during labor.

Are There any Non-medical Reasons for IOL?

- **Social request for personal reasons** — Patients often request for IOL. The reasons include fatigue, sleeplessness, and muscular discomfort as the pregnancy advances, personal choice of delivery date, choice of date after consulting the horoscope and fear of stillbirth (these patients commonly have close friend/relatives with unfortunate occurrences).

- **Favorable cervix** — Some patients are offered IOL when they are deemed "ready to give birth" by their doctor. This commonly involves a routine antenatal consult with their doctor near the delivery date. The doctor performs a vaginal examination and informs the patient that her cervix is dilated and she is ready. This offer is common in modern obstetrical practice. Firstly, as the cervix is ready, the chance of successful IOL resulting in a vaginal birth is good. While the occurrence of stillbirth at term is rare, the consequence is catastrophic. A significant proportion of mature stillbirths remain unexplained. Hence, IOL with consequent delivery allows us to reduce the risk of this occurring.

It is important to note that routine IOL in uncomplicated pregnancies has **NOT** been successful in reducing stillbirth rate and results in higher rates of forceps, vacuum and cesarean deliveries.

Are There Any Risks to an IOL?

As with any procedure, there are certain concerns associated with an IOL. They include:

- **Hyper-stimulation of the womb** — Overly frequent contractions that result from the IOL may reduce the oxygen flow to the baby which manifests as a drop of baby's heartbeat. Some medications may then be administered. However, in unresponsive cases, an emergency cesarean section may be performed.
- **Uterine rupture** — Another potential serious complication is rupture of the womb with expulsion of the baby into the mother's abdomen. This can result in a stillborn or permanent damage to the baby's brain. Fortunately, this is a very rare complication of IOL especially in modern obstetrics. The main risk factors for rupture are in patients with one or more previous cesarean sections and patients who had more than five previous vaginal deliveries (i.e. grand multiparity).
- **Failure of an IOL** — In some instances, the cervix (neck of the womb) remains unresponsive to repeated courses of prostaglandin, and remains tightly closed. In other instances, the labor does not result in progressive dilatation of the cervix. The baby's head may not descend low enough for safe vaginal birth. In rare occasions, the baby is very sensitive to the agents (prostaglandin and oxytocin) used in IOL and responds by manifesting in unreassuring fetal heart trace. In this case,

the infusion has to be reduced or stopped, which consequently may be insufficient to allow adequate power for vaginal birth. When IOL fails, a cesarean section (along with the accompanying surgical risks) is performed to deliver the baby.

As such, an IOL is only performed when the benefits of a delivery outweigh the above-mentioned risks or when your obstetrician is confident that the risks associated with IOL can be adequately minimized by appropriate precautionary measures.

When Am I Considered Unsuitable for an IOL?

IOL is not performed when you are deemed unsuitable for a vaginal delivery in the first place. They include conditions such as a low-lying placenta, breech or transverse lie of the baby.

If you have had one previous cesarean section, an IOL is generally not advised as the risk of a uterine rupture is approximately 2.5%. This is five times higher than the risk of uterine rupture should you go into spontaneous labor on your own, and is considered to be unacceptable by many.

How is An IOL Performed?

Labor starts when the cervix initially soften, shortens and dilates (see Chapter 32). This can be achieved through the **insertion of prostaglandin**, a hormone, **into the vagina**. Locally, the pessary known as **Prostin** is commonly used. Once the cervix is adequately dilated and effaced (thinned out), the **membranes can be ruptured and an oxytocin infusion** (another hormone) can be started to maintain the labor contractions.

1. Prostaglandin application vaginally

Prostaglandin causes softening of the cervix (neck of womb) through a disaggregation of collagen fibers in the cervix. In addition, prostaglandin stimulates uterine muscle activity leading to labor. It is administered vaginally and may be in gel or pessary. Prostaglandin induces the onset of painful uterine contractions which may lead to the opening of the softened cervix. Once the prostaglandin is inserted, the patient is required to stay in hospital for monitoring. The frequency of uterine activity and baby's heart rate pattern are observed.

Women respond differently in terms of speed. The lowest dose regime is commonly employed to prevent over-stimulation. The patient with a favorable cervix has a better chance of responding more quickly. A favorable cervix (determined by the doctor by vaginal examination) is soft, effaced (thin), dilated, faces to the front, with the baby's head well applied and low in pelvis. Some patients may respond with establishment of regular labor pains within six hours; while others may take up to 2–3 days.

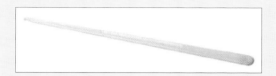

Figure 34.1 Amniohook.

2. *Rupture of membranes and oxytocin infusion*

Once the cervix is favorable, the doctor may rupture your membranes (ROM) followed by administering an oxytocin infusion. Rupturing of membranes involves using an amniohook (specially designed instrument) to break the waterbag (Figure 34.1). ROM alone will induce painful contractions in a proportion of patients. The frequencies of contractions are monitored in the delivery suite and if this is inadequate, an infusion of oxytocin is given to the blood stream via an intravenous drip.

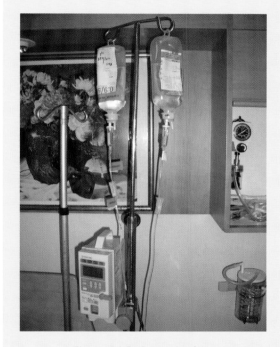

Figure 34.2 Oxytocin drip.

Oxytocin is a naturally occurring hormone produced by the brain that stimulates the womb. This aims to keep the contraction frequency to about four in every 10 minutes. Unlike prostaglandin, oxytocin infusion can be stopped by switching off the infusion. As oxytocin has a short half-life in the mother's blood, the concentration reduces rapidly and this averts potential over-stimulation.

Myths Surrounding Induction of Labor (IOL)

Myth 1.
The patient suffers some pain from the time the prostaglandin is introduced.
This is not necessarily true. Some patients may experience mild pain while the cervix is responding slowly to the prostaglandin. In this instance, she is encouraged to ambulate.

Myth 2.
IOL is 'more painful' than normal labor.
There is no scientific evidence to support this myth. One reason for this perception is that a successful IOL will bring on the labor pains. The inevitable negative association leads to the negative perception.

Myth 3.
IOL is unnatural.
There is nothing unnatural about going through a labor brought about by an IOL. Once labor is established (see Chapter 35), the same rules on progress of labor apply.

Chapter 35

Stages of Labor

Labor is traditionally divided into three stages.
- **Stage 1** — process of dilatation of the cervix which is divided into:
  a. Latent phase — dilatation and thinning of the cervix to 3 cm
  b. Active phase — continued dilatation and thinning of the cervix from 3 to 10 cm (full dilation = 10 cm)
- **Stage 2** — delivery of the baby after full dilatation
- **Stage 3** — delivery of the placenta

The length of labor varies for different women. The average active phase of labor lasts for 8–12 hours in your first pregnancy. Labor is often shorter for subsequent pregnancies.

Stage 1 — Latent Phase

This is often the least painful stage of the labor. During this phase, you may experience very non-specific symptoms such as a mild backache, abdominal cramps, bloody show or passing of the mucous plug. Ambulation can help by distracting you from these symptoms and hasten this phase. You may start to prepare to head for the hospital once the contractions increase or if your water bag bursts.

Duration: variable, from few hours to few days.

Stage I — Active Phase

During this phase, the contractions increase in intensity and frequency, lasting for up to 45 seconds at times. By this time, you should have been in the hospital for an internal vaginal examination to assess the extent of cervical dilatation. You would have been admitted into the delivery suite for the management of this phase of labor.

It is a common practice to manage your labor actively.

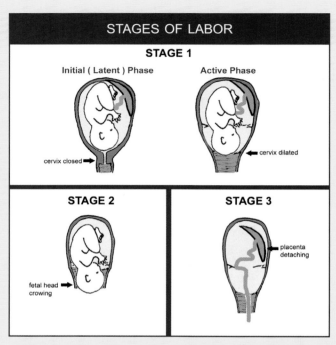

Figure 35.1 A pictorial representation of the various stages of labor.

This entails artificially rupturing your membranes and getting you started on an intravenous medication known as oxytocin to maximize your contractions. Studies have shown that this shortens the laboring process and thus avoids the problems associated with a prolonged labor, such as infections and post-delivery bleeding. Furthermore, the rupture of the membranes enables your doctor to assess the color of the liquor to see if meconium (motion) has been passed out by your baby, which may indicate that your baby is under stress. Be assured that there is nothing unnatural about this as it merely serves to assist your natural delivery process. Furthermore, it does not increase your chance of having a cesarean section.

You will also be offered a variety of pain relief options as mentioned in Chapter 37.

Duration: 8–12 hours (about 1 cm per hour of dilatation).

Stage 2 — Delivery of Your Baby

This is the stage where you are required to work the hardest to help push your baby out. Your doctor and/or the midwives will be beside you to help guide you through this. You may notice an urge to bear down owing to the pressure of the baby's head on your perineum and back passage. This may be accompanied by the passage of faeces but do not be embarrassed. To aid the delivery, your legs may be raised up to allow more room within your birth canal. It is also here that an episiotomy may be made for the delivery (see Chapter 38).

At times, your obstetrician may even need to assist you by using either a vacuum, forceps device or even fundal pressure to help deliver the baby's head (see Chapter 39).

Duration: 30–120 minutes (this may be longer if the clinical situation allows, especially if epidural anesthesia is used).

Stage 3 — Delivery of the Placenta

Once the baby is delivered, your uterus will continue to squeeze out the placenta so that it separates from the wall of the uterus (Figure 35.2). This separation process is usually accompanied by a sudden gush of blood from your vagina. Prior to this, the baby's cord blood will be collected. You can help at this stage by remaining patient while your episiotomy or vaginal tear is being repaired.

In almost all the cases, we do actively manage your third stage of labor. This includes administering an intramuscular injection of an oxytocic after the delivery of your baby, followed by the delivery of the placenta through a controlled cord traction technique. Again, this has been found to reduce the incidence of post-delivery bleeding.

Rarely, separation does not occur and this results in a **retained placenta**. In addition to causing discomfort, it can also give rise to increased bleeding. Under these circumstances, it may be wise to have your doctor ***remove it manually*** by inserting his hand into your womb through the vagina under a general or regional anesthesia (**manual removal of placenta**).

Some patients may opt to claim back the placenta for personal or religious reasons. For others, the hospital would dispose of it in an appropriate manner.

Duration: 5–30 minutes.

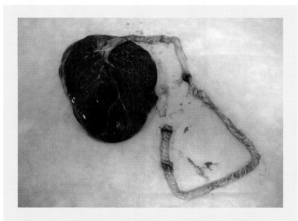

Figure 35.2 Placenta and umbilical cord.

Possible Immediate Problems Following Vaginal Delivery

Immediately after a seemingly uneventful vaginal delivery, some common problems may arise in the immediate postnatal period. These include:

- **Excessive bleeding** due to a poorly contracted womb — requiring additional medication to help contract the womb muscles. You will stay in the delivery suite for a longer period of time after delivery to allow us to monitor you more closely.
- **Vaginal tears** — requiring meticulous repair, sometimes even in the operating theater.
- **Retained placenta** due to a failure of the placenta to separate spontaneously — requiring a manual removal under anesthesia, whereby the doctor has to insert his/her hand through the cervix to remove the placenta.
- **Vulva swellings** — in cases of edema, simple icing is sufficient. In cases of hematomas (blood clots), surgical drainage in the operating theater may be required.
- **Delayed profuse vaginal bleeding** due to remnants of placenta tissue retained — in most cases, this may happen even if the initial inspection of the placenta at the time of delivery had been completed. However, it has been well documented that despite precautionary measures, small remnants of the placenta may still be left behind causing heavy bleeding. Treatment requires admission, administration of antibiotics and medications to help the womb contract. In some cases, an emergency cleansing of the womb may be done in the operating theater.
- **Fever (pyrexia)** — this may be due to urinary tract infection, breast problems (like engorgement, mastitis or abscess), wound/womb infections or rarely blood clots in the lower limbs ("economy class syndrome" or deep vein thrombosis). Appropriate investigations must be carried out so that appropriate prompt treatment can be instituted.

Birthing Positions

Do the different birthing positions like on all fours, squatting and birth stools help in the delivery?

Most women deliver in the conventional ***semi-recumbent position in KK Hospital***. This is a position, which is comfortable for the laboring mothers, especially for those on epidural analgesia. This position also allows the obstetrician to have good visualization of the baby's head position and ease of intervention like forceps or vacuum assisted delivery should the need arise. There is also the rare complication of the baby's shoulder being stuck in the birth canal (shoulder dystocia) after his/her head is delivered. This life-threatening emergency needs the obstetrician to perform maneuvers to save the baby and the semi-recumbent position is best for such maneuvers.

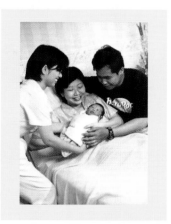

The *"all fours" position*, which is kneeling in bed and leaning forward with support, may help to relieve the back pain when the baby is in an occiput posterior (face up) position (OP) and may also facilitate rotation of the baby's head from OP to occiput anterior (face down) position. Some women use birth balls (of 55–75 cm in diameter) to help them get into the position.

Some mothers may prefer to deliver in the **squatting position** as gravity might assist the delivery process. The use of a birthing chair or stool is recommended for giving birth in a squatting position. However, using a birthing chair has its drawbacks. It may cause excessive tearing of the perineum. This happens when the baby's head puts extra pressure on the perineum. While the tear is not a serious problem, it might lead to more discomfort and a longer healing time.

Unfortunately, there have not been conclusive studies to look into the advantages and risks of the different birthing positions. Thus, it is important to discuss your birth plan and communicate your desired birthing position with your obstetrician so that preparation can be made when you are admitted to the delivery suite. This discussion should commence before you reach term (i.e. 37 weeks of pregnancy).

Water Birth

This concept of delivery involves the laboring mother sitting in a warm tub of water in an attempt to reduce the pain and discomforts of labor in a more "natural" way. Some women who had opted for this have found it a more satisfying method of delivery.

However, there are certain disadvantages associated with it. Some of the hospitals are not equipped with the facilities to support such a birth. Monitoring of the baby's condition becomes difficult with the mum submerged in the water. Infections may also occur as the water is contaminated with urine and faeces. Owing to the warmth of the water, blood loss may be greater after the delivery of the placenta. Great care must be practised to remove the baby from the water immediately after the delivery to reduce other complications.

You should speak to your obstetrician in greater detail if you have any queries over this.

FREQUENTLY ASKED QUESTIONS

1. What is engagement? When do primips/multips usually engage?
Engagement is the movement of your baby's head into the pelvis. It occurs at the end of your pregnancy. Your baby is considered engaged when the head has descended below the pelvic bone. In primips (first time mothers), engagement typically occurs before labor. In multips (those who have delivered before), the baby *may not engage* until the start of labor. During engagement, your abdomen may seem smaller as the baby enters your birth canal. You may also feel some aches or heaviness in your pelvic joints and perineum as well.

2. When does a baby's head usually turn down? If the head is down, will it turn again?
In most pregnancies, babies are born head first. This means that most would have turned to a head down position by 37 weeks. In only 3% to 4% of cases, the babies are found to be *breech* at time of delivery. After 37 weeks, if the baby is still not in a head down position, it is very unlikely that the baby would turn spontaneously.

In some cases, there may be frequent changing of fetal lie and presentation after 36 weeks. This is termed as an unstable lie.

Common causes of unstable lie include:
1. High parity (delivered more than once before)
2. Low-lying placenta (Placenta previa)
3. Excess liquor (Polyhydramnios)
4. Structural womb abnormalities
5. Fetal abnormalities (e.g. tumors of the neck)

In such situations, your obstetrician will need to assess you properly and decide on the best mode of delivery.

Chapter 36

Fetal Monitoring During Labor

> *"The wisdom and compassion a woman can intuitively experience in childbirth can make her a source of healing and understanding for other women."*
>
> **Stephen Gaskin**

Why Do You Need Fetal Monitoring During Labor?

When you are in active labor, your womb contracts to move your baby through the birth passage. The strong contractions may also impair the supply of blood and oxygen to your baby. Thus, monitoring of your baby's condition is essential during this period. Some babies may not be able to handle the stress of labor and your doctor may have to perform a cesarean section delivery.

Monitoring involves measurement of your baby's heart rate at different phases of the contractions. This monitoring may be performed continuously or intermittently.

Continuous Cardiotocography (CTG)

Continuous cardiotocography (CTG) is the most common method used in Singapore. Two transducers are attached via soft straps around the women's tummy. One transducer monitors the baby's heart rate while the other records contractions (Figure 36.1).

CTG is advantageous as ***it detects abnormalities in fetal heart beat patterns early*** so that appropriate measures can be taken if necessary. The main disadvantage, however, is that the woman is "bed-bound".

Occasionally, the transducer at the tummy may not be sensitive to pick up the heart rate well. Your doctor may insert a **fetal scalp electrode (FSE)** to enhance pick up of the baby's heart rate. FSE is a thin tubular device inserted via

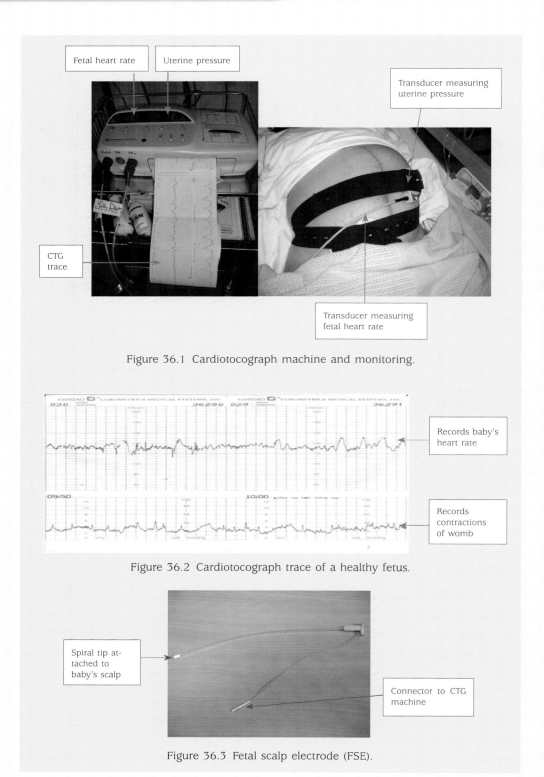

Fetal heart rate

Uterine pressure

Transducer measuring uterine pressure

CTG trace

Transducer measuring fetal heart rate

Figure 36.1 Cardiotocograph machine and monitoring.

Records baby's heart rate

Records contractions of womb

Figure 36.2 Cardiotocograph trace of a healthy fetus.

Spiral tip attached to baby's scalp

Connector to CTG machine

Figure 36.3 Fetal scalp electrode (FSE).

the vagina to be applied onto the scalp of the baby's head (Figure 36.3). There is usually no pain during the insertion (similar to a vaginal examination). The electrode will leave no permanent marks or injuries on your baby's head.

Fetal Scalp Blood Sampling (FBS)

Sometimes, CTG trace may raise suspicions about your baby's condition. The doctor may perform a fetal blood sample to confirm the oxygenation status. In this procedure, the woman lies on her side and a vaginal examination is performed so that a tiny amount of blood can be collected from the scalp of the baby. This is analyzed by a blood gas machine. If the results are normal, labor can be allowed to progress and the process may be repeated again later. If the results are not reassuring, the delivery will be expedited either with a cesarean section or an instrumental delivery.

Some may experience discomfort during the procedure, particularly as it may be repeated more than once. **Many centers *do not* routinely practice this**.

Meconium/Blood-stained Liquor and its Implications

The liquor (amniotic fluid) is monitored throughout the labor. Thick meconium staining liquor indicates that the baby has passed motion inside the mother's womb. This could be associated with fetal distress and the doctor may expedite delivery. There is also a worry that the baby may aspirate (breathe in) the meconium stained liquor, resulting in lung infection and injury.

If the liquor is heavily blood stained, premature separation of the placenta (placenta abruption) needs to be excluded. With premature separation of the placenta, there is an abrupt "cut off" of oxygen supply to the baby and immediate delivery is required.

What is Intermittent Monitoring?

In intermittent monitoring, the midwife uses a Doptone device to measure the baby's heart rate at fixed intervals (every 15 minutes), around the contraction cycle. Contractions are easily felt and the midwife monitors the duration and timing of contractions in relation with the fetal heart rate.

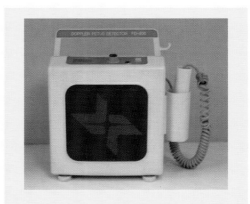

Figure 36.4 Doptone device.

This is commonly practiced either before labor is established or in the early latent phase.

A Healthy Baby in Mind

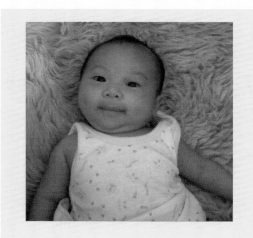

It must be borne in mind that these monitoring techniques are all minimally invasive, in order to be safe for the baby. As a result of the "indirect" nature of these techniques, none of them are perfect. The clinical decisions of the medical and nursing team, based on these monitoring techniques aim to ensure safety of your baby during labor and delivery. After all, delivery is often hailed as the most treacherous journey of our lives and these monitoring devices are safety road marks along the journey.

CHAPTER 37

I Want a Painless Labor

> *Man endures pain as an undeserved punishment;*
> *Woman accepts it as a natural heritage.*
>
> **Anonymous**

As the due date for the birth of the baby approaches, one of the biggest worries facing all mothers is the pain from the labor process. After all, it has been reported that *most* women experience *significant* pain during labor and childbirth.

What is Labor Pain?

With the onset of the first stage of labor, the pain is caused by regular contraction and stretching of the womb and cervix that serves to open the cervix. This stage may last from 8 to 12 hours for first-time mothers. The second stage of labor begins when the baby descends through the birth canal, aided by the mother's pushing. Labor pain is not constant, but increases in intensity and frequency with the progress of labor.

Different women perceive labor pain differently. This perception may be influenced by the woman's previous labor experience, duration of the labor and the use of drugs to accelerate the progress of labor.

What are My Options for Labor Pain Relief?

Childbirth is not a test of endurance. In the age of modern medicine, there are now effective methods for the management of labor pain. Ideally, mothers should seek information regarding these options in the weeks or months before the due date, to allow time for informed decision-making.

Non-pharmacological methods (i.e. not using drugs)

Examples include: hypnosis, hydrotherapy, local heat or cold application, transcutaneous electrical nerve stimulation (also called 'TENS'), acupuncture techniques

These methods vary in their effectiveness but the majority of them have not been proven by studies to be effective. Some of these methods may be useful in short labors. Locally, these methods have not been widely used.

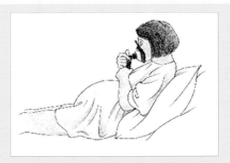

Figure 37.1 Entonox analgesia in labor.

Pharmacological Methods (i.e. using drugs)

Examples include: inhalation of entonox gas, injection of opioids, epidural or combined spinal-epidural analgesia.

Entonox Inhalation

In this method, the mother inhales a gas mixture of 50% nitrous oxide in oxygen, administered via a tight-fitting facemask or mouthpiece. For effective use, the mother should start breathing the gas as soon as contraction begins, so that maximal effect is achieved at the peak of contraction. Entonox inhalation does not eliminate pain but merely alters the mental state so that the pain is felt less acutely.

The effectiveness of entonox in the relief of labor pains varies from individuals to individuals. In general, up to 50% of laboring mums will find this a satisfactory form of pain relief.

Advantages: readily available, does not stay in the body system, and easily administered.

Disadvantages: causes drowsiness, light-headedness and nausea.

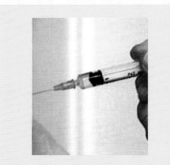

Figure 37.2 Opioid analgesia (Intramuscular injection).

Opioid Injections

The commonest opioid used for labor pain control is **pethidine**. The midwife upon request usually injects it into the muscles of the thigh. Each injection takes about *15 minutes for onset of effect and provides two to three hours of pain relief*. However, it cannot be given when the baby is about to be delivered (usually at least 4 hours before delivery and is limited to situations when the cervix is < 6 cm dilated), as it can cause drowsiness and breathing problems in the newborn. If these occur, an **antidote known as naloxone** has to be administered to the baby to reverse the side effects.

In KK Hospital, devices are available that allow the mother to self-administer short-acting opioid medication into the blood stream intravenously by pressing a button (a technique known as **'Patient-Controlled Intravenous Analgesia' or PCIA)**. This is particularly useful as an alternative for pain relief in *situations when epidural analgesia cannot be administered*, **such as in mothers with bleeding tendencies such as low platelet levels or spinal problems such as prolapsed intervertebral discs**.

Whether injected into the muscles or the blood stream, known side-effects of opioids to the mother include ***drowsiness, nausea and vomiting***. The mother may also have **shallower and slower breathing**.

Epidural Analgesia (EA)

Epidural analgesia (EA) is one of the most reliable and effective ways to relieve labor pain. Pain relief is achieved by the injection of local anesthetic drugs through a small tube into the epidural space within the backbone canal performed by a trained anesthetist.

The Combined Spinal-Epidural Analgesia (CSEA) differs from EA in that an *initial* dose of drug is given into the spinal space, which is also within the backbone canal. This results in a faster onset of pain relief. The decision for EA or CSEA is usually left to the discretion of the anesthetist, as dictated by the stage and progress of labor.

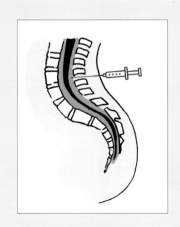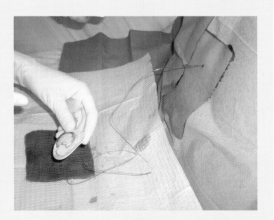

Figure 37.3 Epidural anagesia.

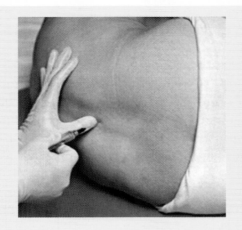

Figure 37.4 Epidural administered while
patient is lying on the side.

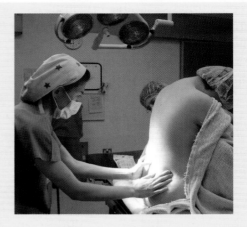

Figure 37.5 Epidural analgesia administered
while patient is sitting up.

*Different positions for administering
epidural*

Although EA/CSEA reduces labor pain
to a great extent, some degree of pain
may still be felt, especially at the time
of "pushing" of the baby.

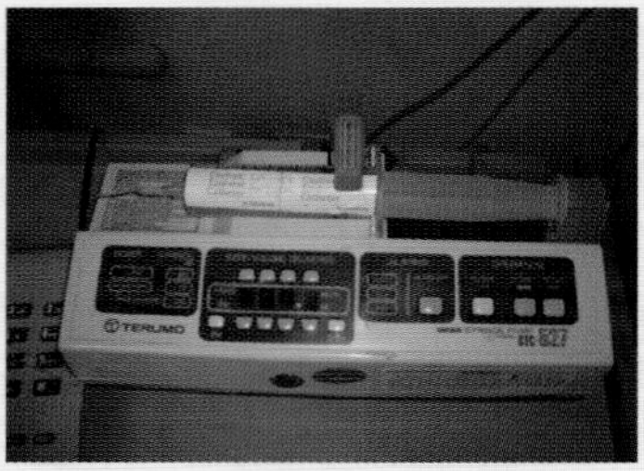

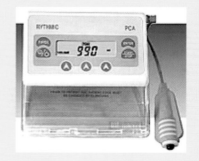

Figure 37.6 Electronic pump
administering opioid analgesia via the
epidural catheter at a preset rate.

Other benefits of EA/CSEA

EA/CSEA can also **help in the control
of blood pressure** of mothers with
high blood pressure in pregnancy — a
condition called "pregnancy-induced
hypertension". As such, it can prevent
the blood pressure from reaching crit-
ically high levels during labor.

**Patient-controlled Epidural
Analgesia (PCEA)**

Figure 37.7 Patient controlled analgesia.

KK Hospital now offers a technique
known as **'Patient-Controlled Epidural Analgesia' or PCEA**, wherein a pre-
programmed device allows the mother to administer additional drugs into

the epidural space by the push of a button. PCEA has greater advantage over conventional EA/CSEA in that the mother has better control over her pain and also uses less drugs during labor.

Myths Associated with An Epidural Analgesia

1. **"There are many side effects associated with an epidural usage."**
   Some minor side effects may occur but they are often minor, transient and self-limiting. These include:

   - **Loss of feeling and muscle weakness**
     Numbness of the legs and lower part of the body is to be expected. The urge to pass urine may also be lost momentarily, but this can be rectified by intermittent drainage of the urine by the midwife. As the epidural drug effect wears out, sensation and strength of the legs and lower body are restored.
   - **Nausea**
     This may result from a lowering of the mother's blood pressure or direct effect of the epidural drugs used. It may be treated with proper positioning and pressure-boosting medicines.
   - **Shivering**
     This may occur although the woman may not actually feel cold. Harmless to mother and baby, it usually does not require any treatment.
   - **Itch**
     Mild itch on the body is more common after CSEA than EA. Usually self-limiting, it does not need any treatment.
   - **Spinal headache**
     There is a risk of a spinal headache of about 1% after EA/CSEA. The headache usually occurs after delivery and is worsened by the upright posture. Medications and a procedure called **epidural "blood patch"** can be used to treat the headache, if severe. In most cases, the headache resolves with time.

2. **"An epidural causes long term backache."**
   Conducted studies have failed to establish a link between long-term backache and EA/CSEA. Backache is common after childbirth, with or without the use of EA/CSEA. Proper back care during pregnancy and after childbirth is important.

3. **"An epidural harms the baby."**
   EA/CSEA does not harm the baby. However, some temporary changes in the baby's heartbeat may occur.

4. **"An epidural can cause paralysis."**
   This is actually ***very rare***. The risk of a permanent damage is actually 1 in 50000–100000. The risk of paralysis is one in a million.

5. **"An epidural can be life threatening."**
   These are actually ***very rare*** and include high blocks, breathing difficulty, convulsions, nerve damage and spinal infection. High standards of medical practice and proper patient selection have contributed to the safety of these procedures.

6. **"An epidural prolongs the labor and increases the risk of a cesarean section."**
   EA/CSEA does not result in a greater risk of cesarean section for the mother. There may be a slightly increased risk of instrumental delivery with an epidural. The benefits of EA/CSEA do outweigh the possible side effects associated with it.

Chapter 38

Pushing and Delivery: Is An Episiotomy Needed?

> There is power that comes to women when they give birth.
> They don't ask for it, it simply invades them.
> Accumulates like clouds on the horizon and passes through, carrying the child with it. "
>
> **Sheryl Feldman**

When you are at full dilatation (i.e. your cervix is 10 cm dilated), you are ready to push and deliver your baby. You may then ask — "To facilitate my delivery, will the doctor make the 'cut' down below"?

What is An Episiotomy?

An episiotomy is often referred to as the 'cut'. An episiotomy is a clean cut with a pair of sterile scissors made under a local anesthetic (so that it is painless) by the doctor or midwife when the baby's head is about to deliver — what is commonly referred to as 'crowning'. This cut is made into the perineum (skin and muscles between the vaginal opening and anus) in order to enlarge the space at the outlet, facilitating the birth of your baby.

What are the Advantages of An Episiotomy?

The main purpose of an episiotomy is to **prevent multiple tears**, which may occur if your pushing is overly fast and strong, or if your perineum is short. A bad, ragged tear is more difficult to repair, and can have healing problems, especially if the tear goes into the anus.

However, even though an episiotomy was done, there may still be a rather extensive tear at times, especially if the pushing was too fast and strong.

Patients in their first pregnancy tend to need an episiotomy more than patients in their second or subsequent pregnancies. This is because the perineum is less elastic and thus, less able to stretch to accommodate the delivering head.

In the past, there has been a belief that routine episiotomies can prevent incontinence, protect the pelvic floor and reduce trauma to the delivering head. However, this theory is yet to be conclusively proven and women delivered without episiotomies seem to do as well as those with episiotomies performed. As such, it is no longer a routine practice.

Nonetheless, there are still a few situations in which an episiotomy may be necessary. These include:

- Your baby's heart rate shows that it is not able to tolerate the last part of the labor well and therefore it needs to be delivered as soon as possible.
- Your baby is big and the doctor or midwife needs some extra room to manipulate within your birth canal so that the baby can be delivered.
- Your doctor needs some extra room to use the forceps or vacuum to help deliver your baby (see Chapter 39).
- Your perineum looks like it is about to tear in multiple places and it is deemed safer to make a single clean cut than to allow the tear to happen.
- You have a rather short perineum.

Types of episiotomy

In general, there are 3 types of episiotomy:

- Midline
- Medio-lateral
- J-shaped episiotomy

In a **midline episiotomy**, the skin of the perineum is cut vertically downwards, towards the anus. In a **medio-lateral episiotomy**, the skin of the perineum is cut downwards and diagonally. In a **J-shaped

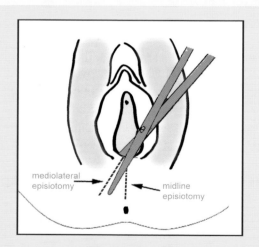

Figure 38.1 Types of episiotomy.

episiotomy, the skin of the perineum is cut vertically downwards before being directed to the left or right.

While both serve the same purpose, there are pros and cons when deciding between the three types of episiotomy. In a **midline episiotomy**, repair, scar cosmesis, post delivery pain, blood loss and healing are more favorable. However, there is a higher chance of it extending posteriorly into your back passage (rectum) and complicating the subsequent repair and healing.

On the other hand, in a **medio-lateral or J-shaped episiotomy**, the cut is slanted away from your anus, thus affording greater protection to your rectum. Therefore, patients with a short perineum will benefit from a medio-lateral episiotomy. Post delivery pain and blood loss may be greater as it cuts through more layers of your perineal muscles.

Only your doctor or midwife can make a judgment at the time of delivery on your need and the type of episiotomy to be made.

Relief of Pain from Episiotomy

In most instances, the after pain from an episiotomy lasts only 2–3 days. This is usually mild and can be effectively relieved by either topical anesthetic cream or oral painkillers. If the episiotomy is more extensive, the pain can be managed with intermittent icing through the help of a physiotherapist. Sitting devices shaped as doughnuts may be used to relieve the pressure on your wound.

Episiotomy Aftercare

The aftercare of an episiotomy is essentially a matter of cleanliness (see Chapter 43). Daily washing with water and frequent changing of soiled sanitary napkins will help keep the wound clean.

Dissolvable sutures are used to repair the episiotomy or tear. These stitches *do not need to be removed* **as they will dissolve within two weeks after the wound has healed**. You just need to keep the sutures as clean and dry as possible. As the area is richly supplied by blood vessels, the wound can usually heal quite well. Passing of urine or stools will not affect the episiotomy. In fact, you are encouraged to ambulate and walk around.

As the episiotomy heals and the wound edges are drawn together, you may feel some mild discomfort. ***Healing is complete after 6 weeks of delivery***. It is essential that you keep to the follow up appointment and after your doctor gives you the go-ahead, you can resume your sex life and exercise.

Chapter 39

Vacuum and Forceps Delivery

> *What seems to us as bitter trials are often blessings in disguise.*
>
> **Oscar Wilde**

What is an Instrumental Delivery?

Instrumental delivery refers to the use of the Vacuum or Forceps instrument to assist the delivery of your baby. Instrumental delivery is actually an aid to facilitate natural birth. Your cervix needs to be fully dilated (10 cm) before either instrument can be used. Your doctor will decide which instrument is more suitable for you and the baby.

How Is a Forceps Delivery Conducted?

Your doctor will gently apply two sterile instruments (forceps blades) into your vagina around the baby's head. The instruments look like curved spoon-shaped

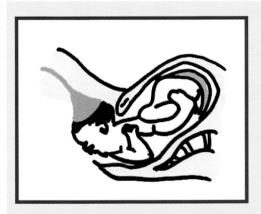

Figure 39.1 Vacuum delivery.

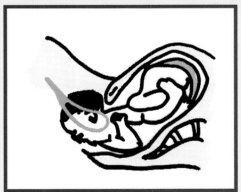

Figure 39.2 Forceps delivery.

tongs, and are specially designed to fit comfortably around the baby's head. As you push during each uterine contraction, your doctor will deliver the baby's head using the forceps blades.

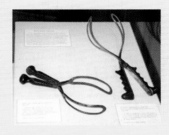

Figure 39.3 Types of forceps.

How Is a Vacuum Delivery Conducted?

Your doctor places an instrument called a vacuum extractor on the baby's scalp. The vacuum extractor looks like a cup. A vacuum is then gently created using a pump. As you push with each uterine contraction, your doctor will gently pull so that your baby's head is delivered using the vacuum extractor. There are many forms of vacuum extractors available but the most commonly used one is the 'Kiwi cup'.

When Will I need an Instrumental (Forceps/Vacuum) Delivery?

There are also a number of reasons why it may be necessary for you to have an *assisted delivery (forceps/vacuum delivery)* during your second stage of labor (i.e. when the cervix is fully opened).

- You are too tired to push effectively to deliver your baby.
- You have been pushing for too long (usually > 1 hour). This avoids the obstetrical complications from prolonged pushing such as excessive bleeding from a 'tired womb' after delivery or a deterioration of your baby's condition.
- The baby's condition has deteriorated and an instrumental delivery would be the most suitable for an immediate delivery. This is usually

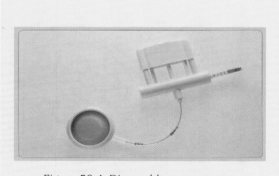

Figure 39.4 Disposable vacuum cup.

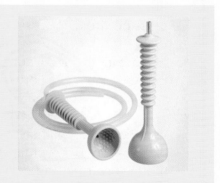

Figure 39.5 Rubber vacuum cup

shown on the cardiotocograph (CTG) that monitors your baby's heart-beat.

An episiotomy may be required when the vacuum or forceps is used.

When Should an Instrumental Delivery be Avoided?

There are actually *very few instances* where an instrumental delivery should be avoided. The following is a list of clinical scenarios where a Cesarean section may be a better option:

- The baby suffers from any rare conditions, such as **bone mineralization defects or bleeding disorders,** predisposing it to injuries or bleeding when delivered instrumentally.
- The **baby is premature** (< 34 weeks gestation) and avoiding a vacuum extraction will reduce more trauma to the scalp and brain. Forceps delivery may be preferred under these circumstances.

What are Some of the Factors to be Considered Just Before an Instrumental Delivery is Carried Out?

There are certain prerequisites that must be present before an instrumental delivery can be carried out.

- In addition to your cervix being fully dilated, your doctor will need to perform an internal examination to ensure that the membranes are ruptured and that the exact position of the baby's head is known.
- The baby's head should have descended low enough into your pelvis to increase the chance of a safe delivery (engaged).
- The uterine contractions must be optimal and if necessary, an oxytocin infusion can be started to ensure this. Your doctor may also apply gentle pressure (fundal pressure) onto your womb to aid in your pushing efforts.
- Just before the application of the instrument, a catheter will be inserted into your bladder to drain out the urine and a local anesthetic drug may be infiltrated into your perineal area to reduce your discomfort.
- The more effectively the mother pushes during the contractions, the less the doctor will have to pull with the forceps or vacuum. This good cooperation and coordination between the mother and doctor increases the chance of a safe delivery.

What are the Complications with An Instrumental Delivery?

It has to be stressed that *most of the assisted deliveries are uneventful* and will be performed with you and your baby's interests in mind. *This will only be carried out if it is felt that you will be able to deliver safely through the vagina.* However, some of the possible problems include:

- **Failure of the assisted delivery with one instrument** — There may be several factors involved. Your doctor will make a re-assessment and decide if you need a cesarean section or if an alternate instrument may be used instead.
- **Complications to the mother** — Pain at and after delivery. Tears or trauma to the vaginal and back passage that may necessitate a repair in the operating theater under anesthesia.
- **Complications to the baby** — Skull fractures or intra-cranial bleeding, potentially life threatening conditions, may rarely occur. Injuries to the facial nerve or eye may happen. During an instrumental delivery, a condition known as shoulder dystocia, (whereby the baby's shoulders may be stuck at the birth canal) can happen and is more commonly seen in bigger babies.

Aftercare Following Instrumental Delivery

If an episiotomy was done, you will need some stitches (see chapter 38). Occasionally, your doctor may insert an indwelling catheter to help "rest your bladder" for a day or two till your discomfort reduces.

FREQUENTLY ASKED QUESTIONS

1. **Which is better? Forceps or vacuum delivery?**
   Although these instruments may be used under similar conditions, your obstetrician will choose the instrument most appropriate to the clinical circumstance and personal preference.

2. **Should I opt for a cesarean section instead?**
   It has to be stressed that *most of the assisted deliveries are uneventful* and will be performed with you and your baby's interests in mind. *This will only be carried out if it is felt that can deliver vaginally safely.* A cesarean section performed under these circumstances may be more risky at a late stage of labor.

3. What will I need to do during an instrumental delivery?

It is important to follow the doctor's instructions closely during instrumental delivery. You should relax and not bear down when the instrument is inserted into your vagina and applied to the baby's head. Similarly, you should push well when asked to do so. This is when you are experiencing a contraction. During a contraction, when you are pushing, your doctor will assist you with the forceps or vacuum to deliver the baby's head. Sometimes, if your doctor attempts an assisted delivery and the baby cannot be delivered safely, you will need an emergency cesarean section.

You would also be required to sign on the appropriate consent forms once the decision for an instrumental delivery is made.

Chapter 40

Cesarean Section

> *When you are a mother,*
> *you are never really alone in your thoughts.*
> *A mother always has to think twice,*
> *once for herself and once for her child.*
>
> **Sophia Loren**

What is a Cesarean Section?

A cesarean section, also called a C-section or LSCS (lower segment cesarean section), is an operation to deliver the baby through the tummy when it is not possible or not advisable to deliver the baby through the vagina. A cesarean section can be planned in advance (elective), or it can be an emergency.

Will I need a Cesarean Section?

A cesarean section is performed either for the safety of the mother or baby or both. Below are some common conditions which may require a cesarean delivery:

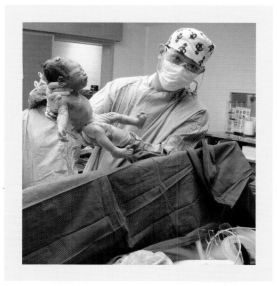

- **Cephalo-pelvic dispro-portion** — The baby is too large for the birth canal and is unable to undergo a vaginal birth.
- **Non-reassuring fetal status** — If the fetal heart rate is persistently abnormal and worrying and threat-

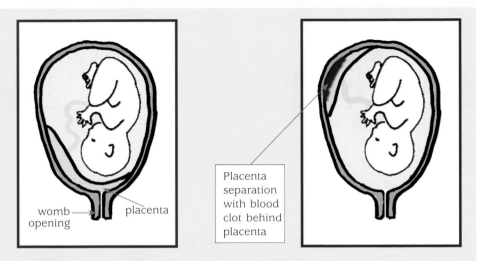

Figure 40.1 Low-lying placenta covering the opening of the womb.

Figure 40.2 Placental abruption (abruptio).

ening the wellbeing of the baby, a cesarean section will be required if vaginal delivery is not imminent.

- **Certain types of previous surgery on the uterus (womb)** — Prior removal of large or multiple uterine fibroids from the womb or multiple cesarean sections (two or more) in the past can weaken the walls of the uterus. A cesarean section is necessary to prevent the tearing of the old wound (uterine rupture) during the laboring process.

- **Placenta previa** — The placenta is low-lying, partially or completely covering the opening into the birth canal, mechanically preventing a vaginal birth (Figure 40.1).

- **Placental abruption (abruptio)** — This is an **obstetric emergency** where there is an early separation of the placenta from the uterine wall before the baby is born. This condition can be sudden and unexpected, potentially endangering the lives of both mother and baby. When abruptio occurs, the mother will often present with a sudden onset of intense and unremitting abdominal pain. This may or may not be associated with bleeding from the vagina. This condition may be very difficult to diagnose in some cases (Figure 40.2).

- **Cord prolapse** — This can occur when there is rupture of the membranes (i.e. "water bag bursts"). The umbilical cord can sometimes slip downwards, below the baby's head, into the vagina. Due to compression by the baby's head, as well as the sudden temperature change, the umbilical cord can constrict, cutting off the blood supply to the baby.

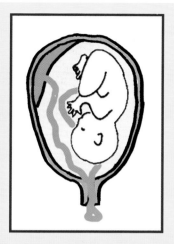 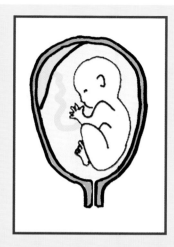

Figure 40.3 Cord prolapse.   Figure 40.4 Breech position of baby
                                                          (buttock down).

This is an **obstetric emergency** and requires ***immediate*** delivery of the baby (Figure 40.3).

- **Malpresentation** — This happens when the baby is in an abnormal position in the womb such that a vaginal delivery is not possible or unsafe. Examples would include a breech (buttock down) or transverse position (horizontal) of the baby. Malpresentation has the danger of cord prolapse when the woman goes into labor and the forewater membranes are broken.

- **Certain maternal conditions** — Some medical diseases may require a cesarean section for various reasons. **In maternal HIV (Human Immunodeficiency Virus) or active genital herpes infection**, a cesarean delivery will reduce the chance of transmission to the baby. In some **uncontrolled medical conditions, e.g. hypertension**, a cesarean section is needed to expedite the delivery so that the underlying medical problem can be treated immediately.

What Type of Anesthesia will I be Having?

There are 2 types of anesthesia used for cesarean section:

- **Regional anesthesia (spinal or epidural)** — You will be ***awake*** during the operation but there will be no sensation of pain from the waist downwards.
- **General anesthesia** — You will be ***asleep*** during the operation.

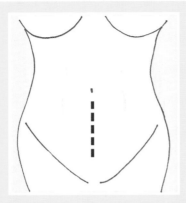

Figure 40.5 Midline skin incision.

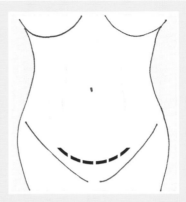

Figure 40.6 Pfannenstiel skin incision (bikini line) — most common incision.

If you are in labor, you can opt for epidural pain relief (analgesia). Should you be unable to have a vaginal delivery and require an emergency C-section, this can be carried out under the epidural as well (see chapter 37).

What does a Cesarean Section Involve?

Preoperative — In an **elective** setting, you should be **fasted for at least six hours**. You will be also be given some medicine to take before surgery to prevent stomach acid reflux. Your pubic hair at the lower abdomen will be shaved. Just before the surgery, a urinary catheter will be inserted into your bladder to drain the urine.

Operative details (simplified description of a cesarean section) — The most common skin incision is a horizontal cut made low on the tummy, near the pubic hairline. This skin incision is often called the "bikini cut" or pfannenstiel incision. The tummy is opened in layers until the uterus (womb) is reached. The uterine wall is then opened, the membranes ruptured and the baby delivered. The umbilical cord is cut, the placenta removed and the uterine wall closed.

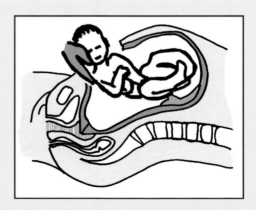

Figure 40.7 Delivery of the baby via cesarean section.

Post-operative care — Depending on your condition, you may be allowed to drink some fluids within a few hours after the operation. Your urinary tubing will usually be removed the next day. You can breastfeed as soon as you are awake and back in the ward. Pain relief will be given so that you can be comfortable after surgery. You will experience some cramps in your lower abdomen as the womb contracts after delivery. For the same reason you will also have some bleeding from the vagina. This is known as **lochia.** Depending on the type of stitches used, you may or may not need to have them removed later.

After a cesarean section, mothers are advised gradual bending and stretching of their legs to prevent deep vein thrombosis ('economy class syndrome'). They are also advised to sit out of bed and start ambulation the next day. In some cases, a leg stocking (TEDs) and/or an anticoagulant to prevent blood clots in the legs may be prescribed. You will need to stay about 2–3 days in hospital after a cesarean section.

Types of Uterine Incisions

- **Lower segment incision** — This is an incision made in the lower part of the womb, and is most commonly performed as it has been shown to have the lowest risk of complications (Figure 40.8).
- **Classical incision** — This is an incision made vertically in the uterus, extending from the lower segment into the upper segment (Figure 40.9). This type of incision may be required for delivery of baby in patients with anterior placenta previa whereby the placenta is implanted into the front part of the lower uterine segment. This incision may also be necessary if there is a large fibroid in the lower segment of the uterus. Such incision is less commonly used as it is associated with greater

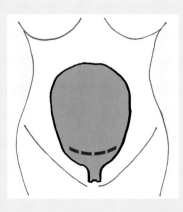

Figure 40.8 Lower segment uterine incision.

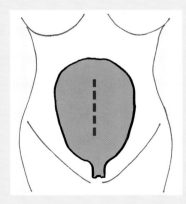

Figure 40.9 Classical uterine incision.

blood loss, post-operative adhesions and infections as well as a higher incidence of uterine rupture in subsequent pregnancies.

What are the Dangers with a Cesarean Section?

- You are *at risk of vomiting* during the operation. If this happens, fluid and food particles from your stomach may pass into your lungs (this is known as **aspiration**) and can cause potentially serious inflammation (known as **aspiration pneumonitis**). Eating during labor may increase the amount of food and fluid in your stomach, and this may increase the risk of aspiration if you have an emergency cesarean section.
- **Though rare, surgical risks are higher than with a vaginal delivery**. These include:
  o   Increased infection or pain in the abdomen (tummy).
  o   Injury to the bladder or to the tube that connects the bladder to your kidneys (ureter).
  o   Removal of the womb as a result of uncontrollable and massive bleeding that occurred during the surgery. (This risk is higher if you have a low-lying placenta or placental previa.)
  o   Developing a blood clot in the legs that may be potentially life threatening (deep vein thrombosis).
- Problems, such as the placenta covering the opening of the womb (placenta previa) or the tearing of the womb, can be higher in future pregnancies.
- Other considerations — Women usually spend a longer time in hospital after a cesarean section (on average, 3–4 days) than after a vaginal birth (on average, 1–2 days).
- Women who have a cesarean section are more likely to have a repeat cesarean section in the future.

Should I Request for an Elective Cesarean Section?

There is now an increasing trend of mothers requesting for an elective cesarean section in order to avoid undergoing labor. Some do it out of fear of a vaginal delivery, while others do it to prevent any perineal or vaginal trauma.

In addition to the possible complications as mentioned above, there are other issues to consider as well. They include:

- A higher incidence of chronic pelvic pain, infertility and dyspareunia (pain during intercourse) after the operation.
- A higher risk of antenatal complications in subsequent pregnancies such as abnormal placenta implantation and scar rupture.

- An increased risk of baby problems such as lacerations and respiratory problems.

In all, research clearly shows that elective primary cesarean section poses much greater risks to both mother and child in the short term, long term and future pregnancies compared to a normal vaginal birth.

What is An Emergency Cesarean Section?

An emergency cesarean section will be advised if it is deemed that you will not be able to deliver the baby safely through the vagina. **The common reasons for an emergency cesarean section include**:

1. A **non-reassuring fetal status** arising during the course of labor and it is deemed safer for the baby if you undergo a cesarean section. A fetal monitor attached to your abdomen may help detect suspicious patterns of the baby's heart rate.
2. A **failure to progress** in terms of cervical dilation and descent of the baby's head. The team of doctors in the delivery suite will monitor the labor progress by regular vaginal examination of your labor progress. Unfortunately in most cases, the failure to progress is often difficult to predict before labor starts.
3. Other special clinical circumstances where it is felt that a successful vaginal delivery cannot be completed safely. In rare circumstances, when an **attempt at instrumental delivery is unsuccessful**, a cesarean section may be advised.

FREQUENTLY ASKED QUESTIONS

1. **If I had a cesarean section before, will I need another one in the next pregnancy?**
   There are pros and cons to a repeat cesarean section and it is discussed in greater detail in the next chapter. However, women who have a cesarean section are more likely to have one again in the future.

2. **Should I undergo an instrumental delivery instead of cesarean section in the second stage of labor?**
   The cesarean section will be performed if it is deemed that you will not be able to deliver vaginally safely. Therefore, your obstetrician will advise on the most appropriate method based on the clinical situation.

3. Will I be able to breastfeed after a cesarean section?

After a cesarean section, women are less likely to start breastfeeding in the first hour after the birth, but if they do start they are just as likely to continue breastfeeding as those who have a vaginal delivery.

4. When is it safe for me to conceive after a cesarean section?

The cut in the womb will heal after six weeks and the womb returns to its pre-pregnancy state. Thus, theoretically, it will be safe to conceive after six months to a year after the cesarean section. However, do take into account the physical and emotional stress of coping with a newborn. Thus, conceive again only when you are ready for the next child.

> **NOTE**
>
> The risk of tear at the uterine scar during labor is not dependent on the period of respite after the cesarean section.

CHAPTER 41

Vaginal Birth after Cesarean Section (VBAC)

> I am only one, but I am one. I cannot do everything, but I can do something. And I will not let what I cannot do interfere with what I can do.
>
> **Edward Everett Hale**

What is VBAC?

VBAC is an acronym for Vaginal Birth after cesarean section.

If I had One Previous Cesarean Birth, Can I have a Vaginal Delivery when I Conceive again?

Women who have had one previous **uncomplicated** lower segment cesarean section (LSCS) and no other problems in the current pregnancy are suitable candidates for VBAC. There are, however, several factors to consider:

- The previous cesarean section
- Current pregnancy
- Other medical or surgical problems

The Previous Cesarean Section

There are again several factors to be considered in the previous cesarean section that was performed. These include:

- The type of cut made on the womb
- The reason for the cesarean section
- Complications that may have occurred at the time of the cesarean section

There are typically two types of incision or cuts made in the uterus during the previous Cesarean section — classical or lower segment (more common) type. A classical incision refers to a vertical cut in the upper part of the uterus. **Women who had a previous classical cesarean section are not suitable for VBAC** as there is a high risk of uterine rupture or tear. A lower segment cesarean section (LSCS) refers to a horizontal cut in the lower part of the uterus (see Figure 40.8 and Figure 40.9). This is associated with a lower risk of uterine rupture or tear compared to a classical cesarean section. Patients with a **previous LSCS may be able to opt for VBAC**.

If the reason for the previous cesarean section is a recurring one such as **a contracted pelvis** (i.e. the pelvis is too constricted to allow passage of the baby), then the patient is **not suitable for VBAC**.

If the previous Cesarean section was complicated by **unexpected tears** in the uterus, your doctor will advise a **repeat cesarean section** in the subsequent pregnancy. VBAC should not be considered in such a case owing to a higher chance of uterine rupture at delivery.

Current Pregnancy

If certain conditions exist that prevent a safe vaginal delivery in the first place, a VBAC will not be suitable. These conditions include a **low-lying placenta** or any abnormal presentations of the baby such as **breech, oblique or transverse lie**.

Other Medical or Surgical Problems

Certain medical conditions such as certain **heart diseases** or **severe high blood pressure** will prevent the woman from enduring the physical stress of a vaginal delivery. **Previous operations on the uterus** to remove large or multiple fibroids may result in weakening of the muscle wall of the uterus. This can increase the likelihood of uterine rupture during labor. In these above-mentioned situations, VBAC will not be suitable.

FREQUENTLY ASKED QUESTIONS

1. **What is the chance of a successful VBAC?**
   The chance of a successful VBAC resulting in a natural delivery may be up to 60–70%. This is generally higher for women who have had previous successful vaginal deliveries.

2. What are the advantages of a VBAC?

As the chance of a successful vaginal delivery is high in properly selected cases, you are able to avoid a repeat cesarean section — thus avoiding the associated surgical and anesthetic risks. In addition, it gives you an option to undergo another VBAC in the subsequent pregnancy.

3. What are the complications associated with VBAC?

The main concern is the ***risk of uterine rupture or tear***. The incidence of uterine rupture is about 0.5% after one previous lower segment Cesarean section, and 4–9% after a previous classical cesarean section. Even if you have had a successful VBAC in the previous pregnancy, it does not negate the existing risks of uterine rupture in your current pregnancy.

Uterine rupture can be life-threatening for both mother and child. It may need surgical removal of the uterus (hysterectomy). **If there is uterine rupture, up to 30% of babies die or suffer permanent brain damage.**

If you desire VBAC and your doctor deems you suitable for this, you will be allowed a short trial of labor. If the labor is not progressing as well as expected, or if the baby's heart beat is worrying, then an emergency cesarean section will be carried out. In most instances, **spontaneous labor is awaited** as there are risks associated with an induction of labor (see Chapter 34).

4. Can I have epidural pain relief if I opt for VBAC?

Yes, you can. There is no evidence to suggest that this is dangerous for you or your baby.

5. What are the precautions for women opting for VBAC?

Women undergoing a VBAC should choose to have the labor conducted in a birthing center where an emergency cesarean section can be carried out within 30 minutes, should the need arise. The need to deliver the baby quickly may occur when there is evidence of possible uterine rupture during the course of labor.

Code Green is a "Crash Code Activation System" when a public announcement within the hospital is used to immediately mobilize the relevant medical and nursing staff to ***ensure the best possible outcome for mother and baby***. **The system, unique to KK Hospital**, is used when time is of essence. A 'Code Green' is for immediate cesarean section when the relevant staff of the delivery suite and operating theater, are activated. This **in-house round-the-clock team of specialists** includes obstetricians, anesthetists as well as neonatologists.

CHAPTER 42

Cord Blood Banking

> *Act as if what you do makes a difference. It does.*
> **William James**

The placenta, umbilical cord and the blood within it is very important in pregnancy. However, the blood serves no purpose after delivery if discarded. Umbilical cord blood is a very good source of stem cells. The blood can be collected after delivery with no risk to the baby or mother. These blood stem cells (BSC) are proven to be useful in the treatment of many blood disorders and cancers.

What Is Cord Blood Banking?

Blood Stem Cells (BSC) from cord blood can be harvested from the umbilical cord after delivery of your baby and clamping of the cord. A small needle is then inserted into the umbilical cord after adequate sterilization. The cord blood with the BSC is then drawn out (Figure 42.1). This process will not hurt you or your baby.

The cord blood is then processed in the laboratory where a specific layer of cells containing the BSC will be extracted. A cryopreservative is then added before placing in liquid nitrogen tanks at approximately -180^0 Celsius.

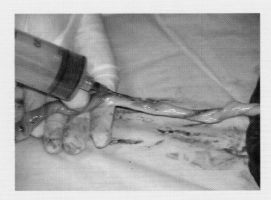

Figure 42.1 Collection of cord blood from the baby's umbilical cord after delivery.

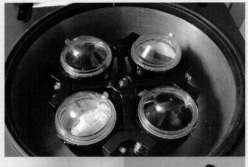

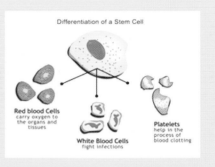

Figure 42.3 Blood stem cells.

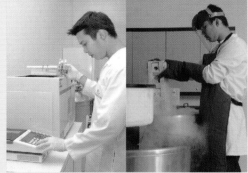

Figure 42.2 Processing and storage of blood stem cells — the cord blood is systematically frozen, minus one degree at a time, to an optimal temperature of –180°C and stored in a liquid nitrogen tank.

What are Blood Stem Cells (BSC)?

BSC are immature cells that are found in the bone marrow and peripheral circulation of an adult. The blood of the umbilical cord (cord blood) also contains large amounts of these cells. They can grow and mature into red cells, white cells and platelets.

BSC are different from embryonic stem cells. There are no ethical issues with BSC as no one is harmed with the harvesting of BSC from the umbilical cord. In fact, these BSC will become waste products if not harvested and stored.

Why are BSCs so Important and Useful?

Since the 1960s, BSC has been used for **stem cell transplants (SCT)**, also called **Bone Marrow Transplant (BMT)** in the past as BSC were harvested from bone marrow. This treatment can potentially cure many diseases, especially blood cancers.

Unfortunately, many patients who require SCT do not have these BSCs. These BSCs are usually obtained from a matched sibling. However, many patients are from single child families (hence, no possible sibling donor) or all siblings do not match in some cases. As a result, many of these patients die.

Can We Use Blood Stem Cells from Anyone?

HLA is Human Leukocyte Antigen and refers to the protein structures on white cells. These proteins are responsible for rejecting or accepting foreign cells. HLA is determined by the genes of both parents. Hence parents and child will only be half matched and the best chance of a match will usually be from one of the siblings. The larger the family size, the better chance of finding a match.

The success of SCT depends on HLA-matching. Graft rejection may occur from a HLA mismatch. Fortunately, BSC from cord blood is slightly different and can tolerate some mismatching.

The importance of having HLA-matched BSC has led to the development of the Bone Marrow Donor Registries from unrelated, voluntary donors in the 1980s. They help desperate patients find HLA-matched donors necessary for life-saving stem cell transplants. The first such registry was the Anthony Nolan Registry in the United Kingdom. It was set up by the parents of Anthony Nolan, who died of leukemia because he could not find a matched donor.

What is Private Cord Blood Banking?

Private cord blood banks started in the mid-1990s as knowledge of the usefulness of BSC became widespread. Individuals who appreciated the value of BSC wanted to store these BSC from their child's cord blood for their own use. This is especially relevant for families who are planning to have one child or a small family size, late pregnancies, and those from mixed marriages. In these families, it may be difficult to find a HLA-matched donor.

Indeed, using your own BSC for SCT may be preferred for some diseases while in other diseases, such as leukemia, it is better to use a matched sibling's BSC.

What is Public Cord Blood Banking?

The first umbilical cord blood transplant was performed in 1989 after cord blood was shown to contain large amounts of BSC. Following this success, public cord blood banks developed across America and Europe and currently, the Singapore Cord Blood Bank has been established here. Cord blood was harvested from voluntary pregnant ladies at delivery. The BSCs were then extracted, frozen and stored. Patients who required a SCT but do not have a donor can then search these cord blood banks for a HLA-matched donor. However, as BSC from cord blood can tolerate some mismatches, it will be easier to find a "usable" donor in public cord blood banks.

Should I Choose Public or Private Cord Blood Banking?

Both banks have their own roles. The public cord blood bank plays an important role for patients in Singapore and other countries to draw upon. Individual families may wish to consider private cord blood banks for their own personal needs.

Discuss with the co-ordinators from both banks to enable you to make an informed decision.

Regenerative Therapy in Future

Regenerative therapy refers to the use of stem cells to produce new cells for treatment of diseased organs. Examples include the use of stem cells for treating heart failure, stroke, Parkinson's Disease, Alzheimer's Disease and spinal cord injuries. However, most of these are still on an experimental basis, but the initial results are very promising!

Common Myths about Cord Blood Banking

Myth	Explanation
"Cord blood collection takes important blood away from my baby."	Cord blood is normally discarded with the umbilical cord after it is clamped and cut. When you ask to have your baby's cord blood collected, the baby's cord blood is collected rather than thrown away. Collections can take place even after the placenta has delivered.
"The cells may not remain viable after long-term storage."	There is no evidence at present that cells stored at −196°C in an undisturbed manner lose either *in-vitro* determined viability or biologic activity. Therefore, at the current time, no expiration date need be assigned to cord blood stored continuously under liquid nitrogen.

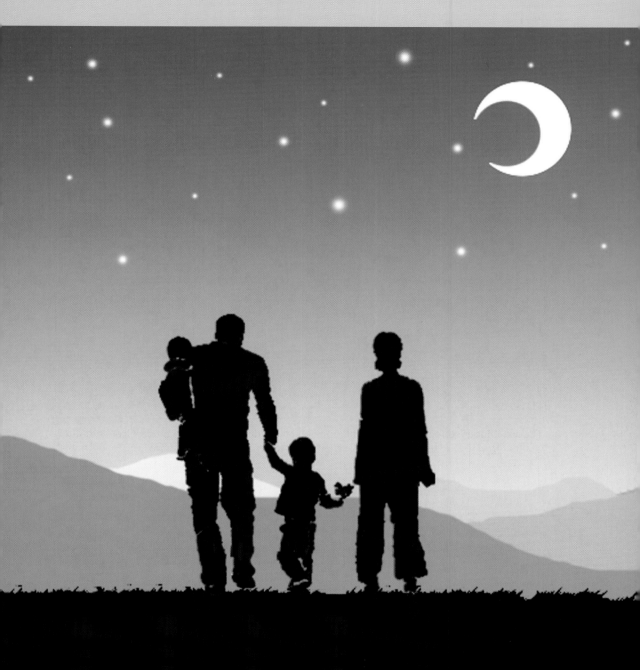

Postnatal Care

Chapter 43

First Week after Delivery: How to Cope with My Wound?

> *A baby nursing at a mother's breast...*
> *is an undeniable affirmation of our rootedness*
> *in nature.*
>
> **David Suzuki**

The wonderful sensation of being a new mum has just begun to sink in, but now your body has to recover fully after the delivery. It is important to know the basics of proper wound care, be it an episiotomy or cesarean section wound.

Care of an Episiotomy Wound

If you had a natural childbirth, it is possible that your obstetrician may have performed an episiotomy (see Chapter 38) for you. Some women also tear naturally during delivery. It is important to know how to take care of the wound so that it heals well with the least discomfort.

To ease the pain and promote good healing of your episiotomy wound, the following can be applied:

- **Icing** — Immediately after the delivery it is useful to apply some ice packs (usually less than 10 mins) to the sore area as this will relieve the pain and help to "numb" the area. It will also help to reduce the swelling. This is usually done in consultation with the physiotherapist to prevent skin damage from excessive icing.
- Alternatively, you can try **perineal ice pad** (e.g. Epi-Kool), which combines coldness and padding. This increases patient's comfort and the coldness is activated by twisting the pad.

- **Good hygiene and wound care**
  - o Keep the area clean after you pass urine or move your bowels by rinsing the area gently with tap water. You can also use soft cotton balls soaked in Chlorhexidine liquid (a gentle non-stinging antiseptic) to gently clean the area three times a day for the first week. There is no need to use strong soaps. Clean gently from front to back to prevent germs from the rectum coming in contact with your wound.
  - o Keeping the area dry reduces the pain and promotes healing. After washing yourself, you can try putting a hairdryer at the low heat setting to dry the area. Also keep the area dry by changing your sanitary pads regularly especially in the first week when the lochia is the heaviest. If you can, expose your wound to air as much as possible.
  - o Avoid sitting for prolonged periods while the wound is still healing. The use of an inflated swimming ring or "doughnut" maybe useful as it relieves direct pressure on the sore area.
- **Pain control** — Your obstetrician would have prescribed you some oral painkillers, e.g. non-steroidal anti-inflammatory drugs which may be stronger and more effective than paracetamol. There are also various anesthetic sprays or gels available which you might find useful.
- **Avoid constipation** — Ensure you have regular bowel movements by drinking plenty of fluids, and take stool softeners, e.g. lactulose or Fybogel for the first two weeks. This ensures you do not become constipated. If you have had a third or fourth degree tear (one which involves the anal sphincter), ensure you keep bowel movements soft with stool softeners. Avoid the use of suppositories or enemas.
- **Sitz bath** — The use of a sitz bath for the first week may relieve pain. A sitz bath is a small basin of warm water with a handful of salt thrown in. You can sit in it, immersing your hips and buttocks and this relieves the pain.
- **Pelvic floor exercises** — Begin doing Kegel exercises as this will promote healing, improve blood flow to the area and improve pelvic floor tone (see Chapter 18).

Care of a Cesarean Section Wound

If you have had a cesarean section, you will need to cope with your tummy wound. Each person's recovery will be different, depending on the medical and obstetrical circumstances and general health of the patient. It is important to remember that it is a major abdominal surgery and you need to take things slowly.

- **Pain control** — To prevent pain from the incision, painkillers will be prescribed. It is likely you will need regular painkillers up to two weeks after delivery. You may also experience uterine contractions, especially when breastfeeding.
- **Early ambulation** — You should get out of bed early and start walking around. This will speed up recovery and prevent the development of blood clots in the veins.
- **Catheter care** — In general, the catheter will be removed the next day after the operation.
- **Suture** — The most commonly used types are the dissolvable ones. At times, you may be asked to return after a week to remove the non-dissolvable stitches or metallic staples.
- **Dressing** — The dressing over the wound may be changed to a waterproof type before you are discharged from hospital. You can bathe but it is important to keep the dressing dry in the first few days. This can be removed after a week. The use of an abdominal binder helps to support the abdominal wall muscles when walking and this reduces pain. The incision wound will feel less painful as the days go by.
- **Breastfeeding** — Breastfeeding can be started any time after delivery.

> ### DID YOU KNOW?
>
> - It takes up to **six weeks** for all your pregnancy related changes in your body to revert back to it's pre-pregnancy state.
> - **Water retention (edema):** You will experience increased urination (diuresis) immediately after your delivery but it may take up to four to six weeks for the swelling to resolve.
> - **Womb (uterus):** Six weeks to return to its pre-pregnancy size and position.
> - **Per vaginal bleeding (lochia):** Takes 4–6 weeks to completely stop. During the first week, the bleeding can be quite heavy but will gradually decrease. It usually changes from bright red to pink or brown, and may become yellow before it disappears.
> - **Episiotomy:** Takes a week for the pain to diminish and up to two weeks to heal.
> - **Cesarean section wound:** Six to eight weeks for the wound to heal.

Social and Emotional Support

Social and emotional support from family members and friends is important. By the end of the sixth week, you should be fully recovered and be able to resume most of your activities. You should ask your obstetrician about beginning an exercise program to regain abdominal muscle tone as well as Kegel exercises for your pelvic floor and when to return for a postnatal check-up.

FREQUENTLY ASKED QUESTIONS

1. **When will my menses return after delivery if I am *not* breastfeeding?**
   Most women have their first menses by ten weeks if they are not breastfeeding.

2. **When will my menses return after delivery if I am breastfeeding?**
   Breastfeeding can delay menses for 20 weeks (five months) or more. However, it is not uncommon to find your period returning sooner or much longer than 20 weeks.

Your Postnatal Visit

At the time of a postnatal review, the doctor will ensure the following:
- You are well and have no problems with fever, urination and defecation or abnormal vaginal discharge.
- You have no breast related problems like engorgement or infections if you are still breastfeeding.
- Your cesarean section or episiotomy wound has healed well.
- Your pap smear is performed.
- Discussing the various options of contraception available and helping you decide which is the most suitable.
- If necessary, your blood pressure will be checked (especially if you had a problem with pregnancy related hypertension) and your oral glucose tolerance test performed at six weeks postnatal (if you suffered from Gestational Diabetes Mellitus during the pregnancy).

Your doctor will decide on the appropriate follow up visits for you after the initial postnatal review.

IMPORTANT

You should see your obstetrician or return to the hospital as soon as possible if you experience heavy bleeding, worsening of abdominal pain, discharge from the wound, wound swelling or fever.

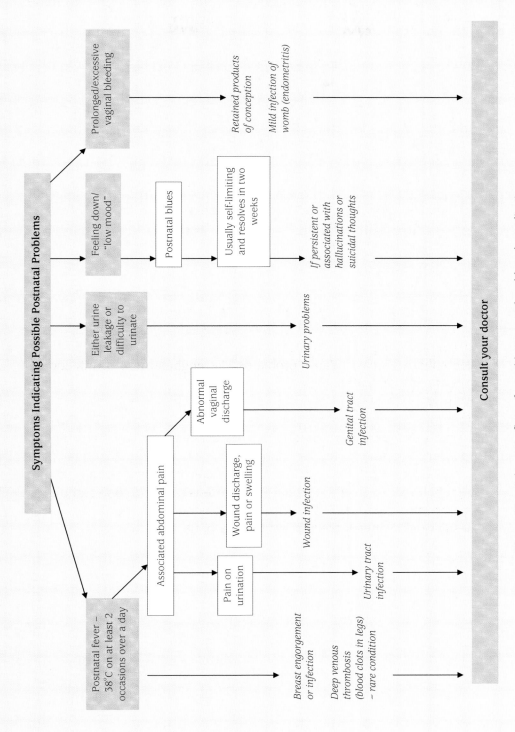

Figure 43.1 Schematic flow of possible postnatal problems/complications.

Chapter 44

Baby Blues and Depression

> The heart of a mother is a deep abyss
> at the bottom of which,
> you will always find forgiveness.
>
> **Honoré de Balzac**

Pregnancy is a special time in the lives of most women. But sometimes, instead of the pregnant or recently delivered woman being in the brink of health, full of excitement and joy, the woman may be struggling with depression.

Let us look into the emotional changes experienced in the period before, during and after pregnancy.

Before Pregnancy

Many women expect to conceive naturally, when she plans to start a family, as will her spouse and their extended family too. This expectancy can itself be stressful if conception is difficult. Some women may then choose to conceive by artificial means, but this can sometimes be even more stressful if the attempt fails. On the other hand, some pregnancies may not have been planned or wanted, and the woman may well be continuing with her usual habits of drinking or smoking or even abusing drugs. All this may later contribute to problems for the mother, such as depression, and for the baby, such as a low birth weight.

Then there are women who already have some form of psychological problems or distress, and perhaps would be on some medication that needs to be stopped for the safety of the baby, whose organs are developing. This may therefore result in the woman being more susceptible to the stress of having to adjust to pregnancy, and later, motherhood.

Keeping in good spirits and physical health is something that goes towards ensuring a good pregnancy. The universal advice of a healthy lifestyle would apply: eating wisely in moderation, avoiding alcohol and smoking, regular exercise, maintaining supportive relationships and participating in a fulfilling activity or hobby. In addition, women and their spouses should make preparations for a new baby, and be mentally prepared for the changes.

During Pregnancy

Many pregnant women describe pregnancy as a glorious time, and glow radiantly, and there is evidence to suggest that pregnancy has a protective effect against some psychiatric disorders.

Sometimes, however, the physical and psychological changes can be so overwhelming, and professional attention may be necessary when the pregnant woman's emotional wellbeing is affected. Some women are much affected by the physical changes, such as weight gain, stretch-marks and morning sickness. Also the idea that hereafter that she will have to be fully responsible for another life, and lose her freedom can be difficult for some others. For the pregnant career woman, sometimes it can be difficult if colleagues are not understanding and supportive. **One in five pregnant women** is likely to have significant depressive symptoms in Singapore.

Those especially at risk for psychological distress include the **teenage mother, single mothers,** those with **previous psychological problems** and those who **abuse alcohol or drugs**. For the first-time mother, the unfamiliarity with pregnancy and life thereafter can make her more susceptible to mood swings. Other factors associated with psychological morbidity include **poor socio-economic status, marital conflicts** or **lack of support**. Then should the pregnancy end either in a miscarriage or abortion, there would be an increased risk of depression as a result of the loss and feelings of guilt.

Some of the disorders include mood swings, anxiety attacks, unusual appetite cravings, and even severe morning sickness (otherwise known as hyperemesis), which can sometimes be disabling.

Antenatal depression

Depression in pregnancy or antenatal depression, is often the first time a woman experiences depression in her lifetime. The common features of depression are also common to the pregnancy state, such as a **loss of appetite, poor sleep, feeling tired and forgetful**. More useful symptoms to look out for would be the emotional features and the negative thinking pattern: easy tearfulness, low mood, irritability, a loss in interest, excessive self-blame and feeling hopeless or that life is meaningless. As mood swings are quite common in pregnancy, one clue to look out for is if these are associated with an **impairment of social or occupational functioning**.

The management of antenatal depression involves looking at the stresses, gathering support for the pregnant woman, and counseling and other forms of psychological therapy. When the depression is severe, especially when associated with suicidal feelings, medication would be necessary, and sometimes even electroconvulsive therapy, which is actually quite safe. The choice of medication must be carefully made, and treatment monitored closely as some of these medications can affect the baby.

Case study

Agnes was a 34-year-old mother who experienced mood swings, loss of appetite and interest and was unable to concentrate at work. She also had excessive self-blame, but did not have any suicidal feelings. The main stressor she experienced was her breech pregnancy, and her worries of the outcome. As she was already in her third trimester, her doctor did not prescribe her medication as it could affect the baby. She received supportive therapy, and her husband was encouraged to spend time with her. Her in-laws, who had mistakenly believed that she was somehow responsible for the complicated pregnancy, were also advised and educated on the nature of breech pregnancy. Fortunately, she had an uneventful delivery by Cesarean operation, and delivered a healthy baby girl.

After Pregnancy

When the baby arrives, many expect the mother will be happy and perfectly at peace with the arrival of the new addition. Also, where she was given special attention and care during pregnancy, the focus is now on the newborn and the new mother sometimes is relegated to being the "milking machine" or "nappy changer". These pressures on the mother can be immense. Her needs are no longer important, whereas the needs of the infant come first. If there is inadequate support and help, especially from the husband, it may be even harder to adjust to the changes.

The **common postnatal syndromes** that can set in include **postnatal blues, postnatal depression and postnatal psychosis**. Others include underlying psychiatric disorders that can worsen with the stresses after delivery.

Postnatal blues

As common as occurring in **two-thirds** of women, the blues hit in the **first week after delivery**, and is **usually short lasting**, subsiding within a few days to weeks. Those affected will feel irritable, weepy and moody. There may be excessive anxiety about being able to cope with the baby, or feeling even frustrated with the baby's crying. Postnatal blues are more commonly seen among first-time mothers who have no previous experience with motherhood, and those with poor support.

As it is usually short lasting, and does not typically affect the mother's ability to care for her infant and her functioning, most mothers with 'the blues' do not need specialist attention. They can benefit with support, encouragement and reassurance from loved ones. Being aware of its occurrence and the normality of having such symptoms is helpful for the woman. However, if you feel that these symptoms persist longer than two weeks, seek further advice from your doctor.

Postnatal depression

Women suffering from postnatal depression often think of themselves as weak or abnormal, but postnatal depression is as common as affecting **1 in 10 recently delivered women**. Typical symptoms include **low mood, irritability, poor sleep, tiredness and a loss of interest in activities. Bodily symptoms such as aches and concurrent anxiety symptoms** are also common, as are negative feelings towards the baby. It is important for the affected woman to seek help, as untreated postnatal depression can affect the ability of the mother to bond with her child, and possibly result in problems in the emotional and intellectual development of the child.

Women at risk of having depression after delivery include those with past psychiatric illness, especially major depression. Those women who were depressed in pregnancy are also more likely to be depressed after delivery. Women who have little support and marital dissatisfaction are most prone to postnatal depression.

Case study

Nancy started feeling depressed and weepy, and tired about two months after the delivery of her first son. She also had difficulty sleeping and had no interest in doing anything much. Although she had eagerly awaited the arrival of her son after trying to conceive for two years, she was alarmed that she felt resentful and frustrated with his incessant crying, and sometimes even had an urge to smother him. Her husband sensed something was wrong, for she had changed from her usual bubbly self, and brought her to see a psychiatrist. She was diagnosed to suffer from postnatal depression, and started on a course of antidepressant medication, with advice to stop breastfeeding. Her mother was roped in to help with the care of her son. And as her mood lifted, she received psychotherapy, which helped her come to terms with her own inner conflicts.

The management of postnatal depression involves consideration of both the needs of mother and the infant. Psychological treatment, or "talk therapy" is especially useful, especially for patients who are reluctant to use medications, or have milder forms of depression. The formal psychological therapies include interpersonal therapy, which focuses on interpersonal relationships, and cognitive-behavioral therapy, which addresses faulty thinking and patterns of behavior.

Some important issues new mothers often feel troubled about are a perceived lack of support or inability to cope with the demands of caring for a child. When the depression is more severe, medication will be required, along with psychological therapy. The choice of medication should take into consideration possible side-effects as well as the individual patient's previous response or particular needs.

Women often fear seeing a doctor, because they are concerned about taking medication if they are breastfeeding. The good news is that there are some medications that are compatible with breastfeeding, so that the mother can continue nursing her baby, for a most beneficial outcome. Sometimes, when the depression is extreme, and the woman has suicidal feelings or thoughts of hurting her child, a period of hospitalization may be recommended, along with intensive treatment.

Postnatal psychosis

This most severe form of postpartum psychiatric illness occurs rarely, at a rate of **1 to 2 per 1000 women after childbirth**. Also known as puerperal psychosis, it usually presents dramatically **within the first two to four weeks after delivery**, with features of **restlessness, irritability, confusion and insomnia. Rapid shifts of mood** are common, from depression to euphoria, and behavior is often disorganized. There may be delusional beliefs, for example, that the infant is a god, or auditory hallucinations that instruct the mother to harm her child.

Hospitalization is required for this illness, which is considered **a psychiatric emergency**. There is a **high risk of self-harm and harm of the infant**. Treatment includes antipsychotic medication, antidepressants or mood stabilizers. Electroconvulsive therapy may also be rapidly effective, and this is beneficial as it enables the mother to recover quickly and return to care for and bond with her baby. Meanwhile, the infant must be put in a safe environment with another caregiver, with the mother encouraged to have contact under supervision. After the mother recovers from the episode, a period of treatment follow-up is advisable as there is a likelihood that there will be further recurrent episodes of non-pregnancy-related psychosis.

Case study

About three weeks after delivering her first daughter, her family noted that Indirah was dazed and irritable. She would frequently look out of the window and mumble to herself, whilst neglecting her baby's cry. In fact, she refused to carry her child, for she believed that he was an evil spirit and he would contaminate her. Her appetite was poor and she refused to bathe for a number of days. Her family finally brought her to the hospital when she was found sitting on the parapet, and she underwent electroconvulsive therapy. Eventually, she made good recovery and was discharged home to be with her husband and baby.

Conclusion

The period before, during and after pregnancy can sometimes be met with various psychological disturbances and disorders. However, with early recognition and treatment, recovery can be good. The goal of treatment is to enable the mother to experience the joy of bonding with her baby.

Chapter 45
Breastfeeding

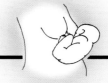

> There are three reasons for breastfeeding:
> the milk is always at the right temperature;
> it comes in attractive containers;
> and the cat can't get it.
>
> **Irena Chalmers**

All mothers should consider breastfeeding their infants exclusively **at least for the first six months** for optimal health and development of the baby. Breastfeeding can be continued thereafter with other foods until the baby is two years and beyond as desired.

Benefits of Breastfeeding

There are tremendous benefits for the infant. Breastfeeding decreases the incidence and the severity of infections, such as diarrhoea, respiratory tract infection and urinary tract infection. Infants with a family history of allergy, who were exclusively breastfed, also had significantly lower incidence of allergic disease.

Breastfeeding is beneficial to you as well! It is well known that breast and ovarian cancer is less common in women who had previously breastfed. This protective effect increases with longer duration of breastfeeding. You will also return to your pre-pregnancy weight quicker.

Mothers who *should not* breastfeed

We would strongly advise that mothers with **human immunodeficiency virus (HIV) infection**, active and untreated **tuberculosis infection** and those undergoing treatment for **cancer**, not to breastfeed. Also, mothers who are on **recreational drug or an alcohol abuser should not breastfeed**.

Prepare for Breastfeeding

Have a breast examination done by your doctor to check for **inverted or non-protractile nipples**. Seek advice from your doctor or a lactation specialist early if you have these problems.

Mother with truly inverted nipples often encounter difficulties latching their babies to the breast. The use of **niplette** as a non-surgical correction of inverted nipples may be recommended during pregnancy from 12 weeks of pregnancy onwards.

Latching Technique

Encourage your newborn to take a large amount of your breast into his/her mouth, with more of the areola and with the nipple pointing towards the soft palate. Hold your breast during the attachment initially and draw the baby to the breast to ensure a good latch (Figure 45.1).

Use different feeding positions such as the football hold or modified cradle hold to facilitate latching on to the breast, as these feeding positions provide better control of your baby's head and achieve a good latch (Figures 45.2 and 45.3).

Increasing Your Milk Supply

Ensure a **good latch** so that there is effective milk flow to baby. Offer your breasts more frequently to your baby. Use **breast compression** during feeding to help increase the intake of milk to your baby. Expressing of milk after

The following is a step by step guide to latching your baby to your breast:

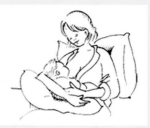

1. Support your baby at your breast level with his body turned on the side and his mouth facing your nipple.

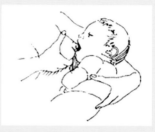

2. Support your breast with four fingers below and the thumb by the side, away from the areola.
3. Tease your baby's lower lip with your nipple to get him to open his mouth.
4. Bring your baby to the breast when he opens his mouth wide.

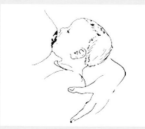

5. Make sure that your baby grasps as much of the areola (the dark ring surrounding the nipple) as possible.

Figure 45.1 Latching technique.

a feed tends to increase the milk supply. *See Chapter 46 for diet or supplements to increase milk flow.*

If necessary, medications such as metoclopramide or domperidone may be prescribed by your doctor to improve your milk supply.

Maintaining Your Milk Supply

Regular breastfeeding usually is adequate to ensure milk supply. You must understand that the milk supply increases with your baby's demand. Avoid substituting or delaying breastfeeding, as this may reduce milk supply because of the reduced stimulation by your baby's suckling.

How Often Should I Breastfeed?

Frequent regular feedings of **eight to ten feeds a day is normal during the initial four to eight weeks after birth.**

Separation of you and baby should be avoided if possible. During separation, **regular pumping** of the breasts (**every three hours**) should be sufficient to maintain the milk supply. The expressed milk can be stored and given to the baby.

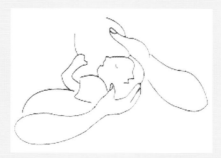

Figure 45.2 Modified cradle hold position — ideal for small infants and newborns.

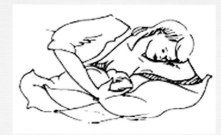

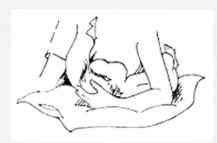

Figure 45.3 Side lying and football positions.

Can Breast Milk Be Stored?

Yes. Expressed milk can be safely stored for up to 4 hours at room temperature, 48 hours in a fridge (at 4°C), 3 to 6 months in a freezer (at −15° to −5°C), 6 to 12 months in a deep freezer (at −20°C).

Is Breast Milk Alone Sufficient to Meet My Baby's Nutritional Needs?

The composition of breast milk changes as the baby grows to meet the baby's nutritional needs. *The World Health Organization recommends that babies be breastfed exclusively for the first six months, and up to two years of age and beyond as mutually agreeable by mother and child*. This means there is no need for other liquids or foods in the first six months, and even after solid foods are introduced at the 6th month, breast milk can be given as the main milk drink.

Managing Breastfeeding Problems

Sore nipples

Sore nipples occurring during the initial few days of breastfeeding are usually due to poor positioning or incorrect latch-on technique. **Correct positioning and attachment is the key to prevent sore nipples**. Seek help as soon as possible to learn the proper technique of latching on.

Purified lanolin cream may be applied to the sore nipples to promote healing. **Breast shell** may be worn in between feeding to protect the sore nipples from rubbing against the clothing. This will also facilitate healing.

Candidiasis (fungal infection)

Candidiasis may present as persistent sore nipples or soreness that appears suddenly with no apparent problems with latching-on. The soreness can be severe with burning sensations or itching, with the nipple and areola presenting as a striking deep pink. You may also notice that your baby may have diaper rash with scalded-looking buttocks and the mouth may have oral thrush presenting as white patches on the tongue and gums.

Please see your doctor urgently, as treatment is required for both you and baby. The infant should be treated with oral nystatin (anti-fungal medication). Treatment of the mother includes topical anti-fungal cream (nystatin, miconazole or ketoconazole cream) applied on the nipple after each feeding.

For persistent candidiasis, oral Fluconazole (Diflucan) may be prescribed for the mother if the baby is at least six months of age.

In addition, pacifier, teats, teethers, breast pump parts, bras or reusable breast pads should be washed and boiled daily. Avoid storing and freezing breast milk during this period as freezing deactivates the fungus but does not kill it.

Breast engorgement

Engorgement occurs when there is a decrease in the frequency of feeding, causing excessive accumulation of milk in the breast. It often occurs during **the first week after delivery** with the onset of the copious milk and especially if there is delay in starting breastfeeding or feeding is infrequent. Apart from the infrequent removal of milk from the breast, incomplete milk removal due to poor attachment can also lead to engorgement.

Engorgement usually affects both breasts, involving the areola and the peripheral area of the breast, which becomes full, hard and tender. If engorgement is not relieved, milk production may be affected. Early initiation of breast-feeding, unrestricted feeding day and night and ensuring proper attachment for effective emptying will help to prevent or reduce the severity of engorgement.

Treatment of engorgement includes **massaging the breast, nipple and areola** area to clear any blockage and to enhance the milk flow. Allow the baby to breastfeed frequently round the clock as the infant suckling is the most effective mechanism for removal of milk.

You can apply a cold pack or cold cabbage leaves on the breast in between feeding to help reduce swelling, warmth and pain. Take analgesia medication such as Paracetamol to alleviate the pain.

Apply warm packs only if the breasts are leaking after the breast massage as the heat from the warm packs may aggravate the swelling if the ducts are blocked. Seek help from a lactation specialist if engorgement is not relieved with the above measures.

Plugged ducts

A plugged duct is a localized blockage of milk resulting from milk stasis. It usually presents as a **painful palpable lump** with well-defined margins. It may be caused by inadequately drainage in one area of the breast or by tight or restrictive clothing. Plugged ducts can develop into mastitis if not treated adequately.

Massaging the breast is an effective way to help dislodge the blocked milk. Continue to breastfeed and commence feeding on the affected breast to promote drainage. Massage the affected breast before and during feeding to stimulate the flow of the milk. **Apply warm compress** to the affected area before feeding once the milk starts to leak after the massage. **Use different feeding positions** to help drain the different parts of the breast. Seek medical advice if redness and fever are present as **antibiotics may be indicated**.

Milk blister

Milk blister is a whitish, tender area, often found at the tip of the nipple. It seals a nipple pore preventing the duct system from draining and causing milk buildup behind the occlusion. This leads to a blocked milk duct.

Breast massage should be done to clear the build up of milk. Continue breastfeeding to clear the blocked milk duct. Seek help from a doctor or a lactation specialist, as it may be necessary to break the skin using a sterile needle.

Mastitis

Mastitis refers to a unilateral bacterial infection of the breast. It may cause **fatigue, localized breast tenderness and a flu-like, muscular aching with fever**. The infection, which is usually unilateral, is located in one area of the breast. Stress, fatigue, cracked nipples, plugged ducts, a tight bra, engorgement and an abrupt change in the feeding frequency can predispose to mastitis.

Treatment of mastitis includes **massaging the breast** to clear the plugged ducts. **Apply moist heat** to promote drainage once milk is leaking after massage. You can continue to breastfeed. Increase your intake of fluids and take antipyretics to reduce fever. See your doctor early for antibiotic therapy.

Breast abscess

Mastitis may develop into abscess (collection of pus) if the treatment is delayed or inadequate. **Breastfeeding can be continued on the unaffected breast**. Continue to **hand-express or pump the milk from the affected breast** to prevent engorgement and to maintain milk supply.

Fine-needle aspiration under ultrasound guidance or incision and drainage could be done by your doctor to drain the pus.

FREQUENTLY ASKED QUESTION

1. **Can I continue to breastfeed my baby if I am pregnant again?**

   There are a few concerns about continuing breastfeeding during pregnancy. Firstly, there is the **concern about deficiency of nutrients** to the developing fetus and the impact on the mother's health such as depleting her own store of calcium. Thus, continue to take prenatal vitamins and calcium supplements as well as continue a healthy diet. Secondly, the pregnancy hormones may also **decrease the amount of milk as well as change the taste of the milk**.

There are some studies which link breastfeeding to miscarriage and premature labor although the results were not conclusive. **If you are experiencing these symptoms, do inform your doctor.**

2. **Is it normal if I start leaking milk at seven months of pregnancy?**
   The milk glands in your breasts may start to produce colostrum as early as seven months of pregnancy. Thus, it is not unusual if your breasts leak colostrum at this stage.

3. **I notice an extra breast tissue in the armpit. Is this normal?**
   Some women may have an extra breast or pair of breasts in the lower armpit, known as **accessory breasts**. These extra breasts may also enlarge due to hormonal stimulation in pregnancy. So, do not be alarmed.

4. **Can I breastfeed if I have had breast augmentation surgery with implants?**
   Many women who have have had breast augmentation or implants ask if they can breastfeed. For most women, breastfeeding is no more difficult with implants than without.

   For women who have silicone implants, there is the fear that breastfeeding would endanger the child. However, studies have shown **no adverse effects** as the silicone molecule is too large to pass into the milk ducts. Nowadays, silicone implants have been replaced by saline implants. Even if the saline leaks into the milk, there will not be any harmful effects on the baby as saline is an inert substance.

Chapter 46

Eating Right for Breastfeeding

> A newborn baby has only three demands. They are warmth in the arms of its mother, food from her breasts, and security in the knowledge of her presence. Breastfeeding satisfies all three.
>
> **Grantly Dick-Read**

When you are breastfeeding your baby, you must continue to eat well to maintain your nutritional status. Your nutrient stores may be used up for breast milk if your nutrient intake is low. In fact, your requirement for certain nutrients (e.g. energy, protein and B vitamins), are higher during breastfeeding than during pregnancy. So if you were conscious of the nutritional quality of your diet during pregnancy, there is even more reason for you to do so when breastfeeding!

In general, if you eat a balanced diet based on the 'Healthy Diet Pyramid for Pregnancy' (see Chapter 25), you will be able to meet your basic nutritional needs during breastfeeding in order to support your baby's growth and development, as well as protect your own nutrient stores. Eat whenever you are hungry and drink when thirsty.

Special Formulated Milks for Breastfeeding Mothers

Most special milks formulated for breastfeeding mothers are based on powdered skimmed or whole cow's milk, fortified with specific vitamins and minerals, especially iron, zinc and B vitamins including folic acid. Some brands also contain fish oil, as a source of DHA (Docosahexaenoic acid). Hence, breastfeeding mothers who are unable to consume a balanced diet consisting of the recommended number of servings of meat (as main source of iron and zinc), citrus fruits and green leafy vegetables (as main sources of folic acid), and cold water deep-sea fishes (as main source of DHA) may benefit from drinking these special milks to supplement their usual sources of these nutrients. However, the basic nutrients, namely, calcium, phosphorus and protein, found in special milks formulated for breastfeeding mothers and regular milk are similar.

Caffeine and Breastfeeding

As caffeine passes from mother to baby through breast milk, excessive caffeine can cause symptoms of caffeine stimulation in your baby. Regular coffee drinkers would be glad to know that one or two cups of coffee a day will not affect babies as studies suggest that breastfeeding mothers can consume up to 650 mg of caffeine a day. However, be aware that apart from coffee, tea and cocoa products, caffeine can also be found in soft drinks and over-the-counter medications like cold medicines.

Avoid Alcoholic Beverages When Breastfeeding

Alcohol passes from mother to baby through breast milk. Large amounts of alcohol can affect the milk let-down (ejection) reflex. Most local lactation experts recommend that mothers refrain from drinking alcoholic beverages in the first week after delivery to avoid stressing the newborn baby's liver. However, from the second week onwards, if baby is not jaundiced, and mother wishes to consume alcohol, she should not exceed 0.5 g alcohol for every kilogram of body weight, and breastfeeding should be delayed for at least one hour for every 10 g of alcohol consumed. (***One pint of beer, one glass of wine or one standard drink of spirits is equivalent to one unit of alcohol. This equals 10 g of alcohol.***)

Case example

A 60 kg woman can drink a maximum of 0.5 g × 60 = 30 g (namely, 3 units) of alcohol a day. If she chooses an alcoholic drink containing 20 g of alcohol, she should wait at least two hours before breastfeeding her baby.

DID YOU KNOW?

- Benedictine Dom™, an alcoholic tonic traditionally associated with good health and consumed by mothers post-delivery contains about 40% alcohol. So, 25 ml of Benedictine DOM would be equivalent to 10 g of alcohol (one unit).

- Alcohol added to food during cooking does evaporate, but some alcohol will still be left. So, if you are eating dishes cooked in alcohol, for example, red wine chicken, you may wish to refrain from breastfeeding your baby for the next 1–2 hours.

Table 46.1 Caffeine content in different beverages.

Beverage	Caffeine content	Comments
Instant coffee	60–100 mg per cup	The amount of caffeine depends on how much you put in the cup. one rounded teaspoon of instant coffee powder contains 47 mg of caffeine.
Fresh coffee	80–350 mg per cup	The amount of caffeine depends on the type of beans, the way the coffee is made and strength of the brew.
Decaffeinated coffee	2–4 mg per cup	1 rounded teaspoon of decaffeinated instant coffee powder contains 2 mg of caffeine.
Tea	8–90 mg per cup	Caffeine content depends on strength of brew.
Cola drinks	35 mg per 250 ml serving	
Cocoa and hot chocolate	10–70 mg per cup	The amount of caffeine depends on how much you put in the cup.
Chocolate bars	20–60 mg per 200 g bar	
Some prescription and over-the-counter medications	20–100 mg per dose	Some medicines (cough and headache medicines) contain caffeine.

FREQUENTLY ASKED QUESTIONS

1. **Do I need to avoid certain food (for example, eggs, cow's milk, fish, nuts or wheat) to reduce my baby's risk of developing allergies?**
   There is not enough evidence currently that avoiding specific foods will reduce baby's risk of developing allergies. However, if there is a family history of allergy, some doctors may recommend delaying the introduction of certain foods, e.g. eggs, cow's milk and nuts, till the baby is older. You may wish to consult your doctor for more advice when baby is six months old and ready to start solid foods.

2. **Does eating ginger cause my baby to be jaundiced if I breastfeed?**
   There is no evidence that ginger or any foods consumed by the breastfeeding mother will cause baby to be jaundiced. Jaundice is due to the accumulation of bilirubin in the baby's body. Bilirubin is a by-product of red blood cell breakdown, which occurs naturally every day. However, as the newborn baby's liver is immature, bilirubin breakdown is slow, hence leading to accumulation and the characteristic yellow coloration of baby's skin and eyes.

3. **Is it safe to consume artificially sweetened foods and drinks when breastfeeding?**

Moderate consumption of approved sweeteners like aspartame, acesulfame potassium and sucralose is considered safe when breast feeding. These sweeteners are used as table top sweeteners, e.g. Equal™, Palsweet™, are used by food manufacturers in low calorie products like drinks, yoghurts and confectionaries.

4. **Can I go on a weight loss diet without affecting my breast milk supply?**

Most breastfeeding mothers will lose their weight gained during pregnancy. Losing 1 to 2 kg a month is considered as healthy weight loss. Going on a weight loss diet whilst breastfeeding is not recommended as you may not be consuming enough nutrients to meet your requirements, and breast milk production may be affected. Use your weight as an indicator — if you are losing more than 2.5 kg a month after the first month, you may be eating too little.

5. **Is there any special diet to increase breast milk production?**

Traditional foods such as unripe papaya cooked with fish has been advocated to increase mother's milk.

Fenugreek, also known as 'venthaiyem' (in Tamil), 'methi' (in Hindi) or 'Halba' (in Malay) is the herb that is commonly used in cooking curry. It has been used to increase milk supply traditionally.

Fenugreek tea can be taken four times a day by adding three teaspoons of fenugreek seeds into a glass of hot water to improve milk supply. Fenugreek capsules are available from health food outlets and pharmacies and can be taken as two capsules four times a day or three capsules three times a day to improve milk supply.

Fenugreek is considered safe for nursing moms when used in moderation and is listed as GRAS (Generally Recognized As Safe) by US FDA. However, be cautious that an excessive amount of fenugreek may cause loose stools in the mother. See Table 46.2 for medication to increase milk flow.

Table 46.2 Medication to increase milk flow

Medication	Dose	Comments
Domperidone	10 mg thrice a day	For ten days
Metoclopramide	10 mg thrice a day	For ten days

Chapter 47

Feeding Your Baby: Breast or Bottle?

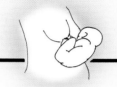

> *It is only in the act of nursing that a woman realizes her motherhood in visible and tangible fashion; it is a joy of every moment.*
>
> **Honore de Balzac**

Breastfeeding gives your baby the best start to his/her life. Breastfeeding is the most natural way of feeding and is also the best source of nutrition for your baby. The nutritional composition of breast milk changes according to your baby's needs which can vary, from day to day, and during the day.

Colostrum — The First Milk

Colostrum is the first milk, which is produced for the first few days after birth. Its composition is very different from mature breast milk. It is important for the baby's long-term health and development.

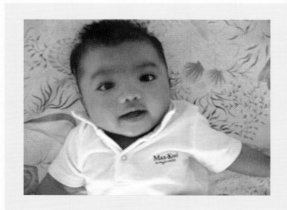

Colostrum has a higher content of protein than mature breast milk. Much of the protein is present as immunoglobulins (antibodies), which help to protect your baby against infection. Also, colostrum has a lower fat content than mature milk and is rich in minerals and vitamins A, D and B12.

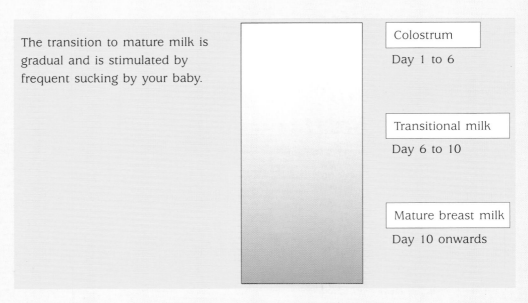

The transition to mature milk is gradual and is stimulated by frequent sucking by your baby.

Colostrum

Day 1 to 6

Transitional milk

Day 6 to 10

Mature breast milk

Day 10 onwards

Figure 47.1 Composition of mature breast milk.

Energy

The energy requirements of infants reflect the amount needed to promote health, adequate growth, optimal body composition and levels of physical activity appropriate for their developmental age. On the per weight basis, infants require 3–4 times more energy than adults.

The energy in breast milk is provided by fats, carbohydrates and proteins in the following proportions:

Fat

Fat is a concentrated source of energy, which is needed for growth and development. Fat also provides the infant with a source of essential fatty acids and long chain polyunsaturated fatty acids (LCPs), DHA for brain, retina and nervous tissue development and is necessary for the absorption of the fat-soluble vitamins A, D, E and K.

The fat content of breast milk is highly variable. It varies during a feed (more fat in hind milk) and at different times of the day (lowest fat in early morning).

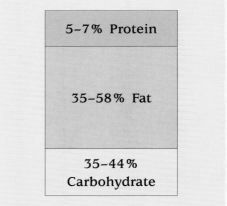

5–7% Protein

35–58% Fat

35–44% Carbohydrate

Figure 47.2 Composition of breast milk.

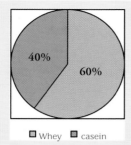

Whey and casein provides protein for growth and development. The ratio of 60:40 in breast milk allows for quick and easy digestion.

Figure 47.3 Protein composition of mature breast milk.

Carbohydrate

Carbohydrates provide infants with a major source of energy, freeing protein for growth. The main carbohydrate source in breast milk is lactose. Lactose is beneficial for the baby as it enhances calcium absorption.

Breast milk also contains a group of non-digestible carbohydrates called oligosaccharides. Oligosaccharides are not digested in the upper part of the gastro-intestinal tract, reaching the colon intact. Here, they are used as food for the beneficial bacteria (e.g. Bifidobacteria) present in the intestine and increasing their numbers. Bifidobacteria has been shown to have protective properties such as inhibition of pathogens (disease forming bacteria) as well as supporting the development of the immune system.

Protein

Protein provides infants with a source of essential amino acids for growth. Breast milk contains two types of protein, **whey** and **casein**.

However, excess protein may put unnecessary stress on the immature kidneys of baby.

Summary of the Important Roles of Breast Milk

Roles	Breast milk constituents (Examples only, not complete list)
Energy and growth	Fat, carbohydrates, protein, growth factors, nucleotides
Brain and eye	LCPs, taurine
Digestive system	Oligosaccharides, taurine, enzymes
Immune system, defence	Immunoglobulins, selenium, beta-carotene, nucleotides, oligosaccharides
Cardiovascular system and blood	Iron, lactoferrin, vitamin K
Bones	Calcium, phosphorus, vitamin D

Bottle-feeding Your Baby

While breast milk is superior for the newborn baby, infant milk formula plays an important role in infant nutrition when breast milk supplementation is required. The search for breast milk substitutes has been conducted for centuries. Many advances have been made to bring the composition of infant formula milk closer to breast milk. Important modifications have included reduction in protein content, addition of vitamins, trace elements and lactose and alteration of the whey:casein ratio. The final aim is not necessarily to mimic the composition of breast milk in every respect, but to achieve the functional benefits of breast milk.

All infant milk formulas that are available in the market today are formulated in accordance to the Codex Alimentarius standards. They are safe and nutritionally adequate for feeding your baby.

According to the World Health Organization, there are exceptional circumstances in which a mother can be considered to be unable to breastfeed her baby; for example, if the mother has a chronic illness (such as HIV infection or tuberculosis) or is under certain medication. If you have decided to bottle feed your baby, you will have to start by selecting the right infant milk formula. Your doctor can help you pick one based on your baby's needs.

Why Infant Milk Formula Instead of Cow's Milk?

Many parents wonder why they cannot just feed their baby regular cow's milk.

The answer is simple: young babies cannot fully digest this product as completely or easily as they digest formula. Also, cow's milk contains high concentrations of protein and minerals, which can stress a newborn's immature kidneys and cause dehydration.

In addition, this feeding lacks the proper amounts of iron and vitamin C that infants need. It may even cause iron-deficiency anemia in some babies, since protein can irritate the lining of the stomach and intestines, leading to loss of blood into the stools. For these reasons, your baby should not receive any regular cow's milk for the first year of life.

Choosing An Infant Milk Formula

When shopping for a manufactured infant formula, you will find **three basic types**:

- **Cow's milk-based formulas** account for about 80% of the formula sold today. Though cow's milk is at its foundation, the milk has been changed dramatically to make it safe for infants. It is treated by heating and other methods to make the protein more digestible and less potentially allergenic. More milk sugar (lactose) is added to make the concentration equal to that of breast milk, and the fat (butterfat) is removed and replaced with vegetable oils that are more easily digested by infants.

Cow's milk infant formulas are fortified with iron. If your baby is full-term, he should have enough natural reserves of iron to meet his needs for his first four to six months. After six months, however, he needs some extra iron in his diet, and iron-fortified formula is one way to meet this requirement.

- **Soy formulas** contain a different protein (soy) and different carbohydrate (glucose polymers or sucrose) from milk-based formulas. They are recommended as an alternative for babies who are unable to digest lactose, the main carbohydrate of cow's milk formula.

  If you choose to use soy products, be sure to use a soy-based infant formula — not regular soymilk.

- **Specialized formulas** are manufactured for infants with particular disorders or diseases. Protein hydrolysate formulas are meant for babies who have a family history of milk allergies. It is easier to digest and less likely to cause allergic reactions than standard cow's milk formula because the proteins are broken down.

  There are other specialized formulas, such as those for infants with low birth weight, problem of regurgitation, inability to digest fat and other conditions. There are also formulas made specifically for premature babies. If your newborn has special needs, consult your pediatrician on which formula is best for your baby.

Preparation of Infant Formula

Infant formulas are available in ready-to-feed liquid forms or as powders. Powders are available either as pre-measured individual packets or in a can with a measuring scoop. To prepare it, each scoop of powdered formula must be mixed with the specified amount of water.

It is important to follow the manufacturer's directions exactly. Do not pack the scoop with too much of powder as this will increase the concentration of the feed. Adding the right amount of water is also important. If you add too much water, your baby would not get the calories and nutrients he/she needs for proper growth; and if you add too little water, the high concentration of formula could cause diarrhoea or dehydration and will give your baby more calories and nutrients than he needs.

Whichever type of infant formula you choose, proper preparation and refrigeration are essential.

Remember that no infant milk formula can surpass breast milk as the ideal and unique food for healthy term infants. Continuous research is still in progress to identify the role of different substances in breast milk so that the breast milk benefits can be integrated into infant milk formulas.

Chapter 48

Returning to Pre-Pregnancy Weight and Shape

> *Never, never, never quit.*
>
> **Winston Churchill.**

After delivery, many of the physical changes of pregnancy will persist for four to six weeks. Resuming pre-pregnancy exercises should be gradual and varied according to the individual.

Exercise Regime

You should aim to exercise for at least three times a week, with each session lasting for 30 minutes. Do make sure that you have at least 5 to 10 minutes of warm up and cooling down (see Chapter 16).

Exercise and Breastfeeding

It is ideal that you breastfeed before you exercise to avoid the build up of lactic acid in the breast milk. Adequate nutrition and hydration are important before you start your exercise. Moderate weight loss for the mother is safe at this stage. Aim for 1–2 kg of weight loss a month. Excessive weight loss may lead to decrease in milk production.

Recommended Types of Exercises

- **For first 6 weeks after delivery**
Walking
Abdominals — tummy exercise and curl up **(Avoid if you had a Cesarean Section)**
Pelvic tilt
Pelvic floor muscle exercise (see Chapter 18)

- **After 6 weeks of delivery**

Walking

Swimming

Low impact aerobics

Pilates

Yoga

Fitball

Aqua exercise

Abdominals — curl up and obliques

- **After 4 months of delivery**

Sports

Jogging/running

Moderate to high impact aerobics

With regular exercise, proper diet and breastfeeding, it will be a breeze before you return to your pre-pregnancy weight and shape!

Chapter 49

Care of the Newborn

> The hand that rocks the cradle may not rule the world, but it certainly makes it a better place. '
>
> **Margery Hurst**

Your new baby's appearance will probably be a surprise to you. They may have wrinkly skin and be covered in a white, greasy substance called **vernix caseosa**. Their head shape may look squashed on one side and their eyes puffy because of the pressure of passing through the birth canal. All this will usually disappear in time.

Take your baby in your arms as soon as possible and you all can start to bond.

Do not forget that your baby has already been listening to your voices for the past few months, and he/she will feel reassured listening to it again now, when in this new environment. Mums should try and establish breastfeeding as soon as possible. This will stimulate the flow of milk and enhance bonding.

Newborn babies vary in how much they weigh and how long they are. Average weight of a baby ranges from 2.5 kg to 3.5 kg, length from 45 to 54 cm and head circumference is from 32 to 36 cm.

Your baby's doctor will usually check your baby within the first day of life. They will do a thorough examination, checking the growth as well as looking for abnormalities such as **heart defects**, **eye abnormalities**, **developmental dysplasia of the hip**, **undescended testes** (if you have a boy) and other conditions.

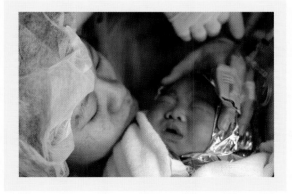

Newborn Screening

- Newborn screening is done to check your child for health problems.
- These conditions could prevent permanent damage or even death if detected early.
- **In Singapore, newborns are screened for**
    - o   G6PD deficiency (lack of an enzyme)
    - o   Hypothyroidism (low thyroid function)
    - o   Hearing loss
    - o   Metabolic Disease (looking for Inborn Errors of Metabolism, which are disorders involving abnormalities in the breakdown of fats or proteins)

Common Skin Conditions

During the first few weeks, your baby will usually have a few of the common skin conditions.

- **Milia:** Small white dots that usually appear on baby's nose and chin. They are the result of immature sweat glands and will disappear in time without any treatment.
- **Erythema toxicum**: This is a red rash with a raised white center that looks like pimples. They can appear anywhere on the baby's body and tends to come and go within the first few weeks of the baby's life. They too will disappear without treatment. The baby is very well with it, but as this rash can be confused with more serious rashes, it is best to check with your doctor.
- **Seborrhoeic dermatitis (Cradle cap):** This is dry flaky skin on the scalp, eyebrows and occasionally behind the ears. Massaging in some baby oil/olive oil will help soften the flakes.
- **Diaper rash**: This occurs due to the ammonia and other chemicals in the urine/feces. It is advisable to apply a protective emollient or barrier cream at each diaper change. If the rash does not improve, see your doctor as it could be thrush, which is caused by a fungus and would require medication to improve.
- **Dry skin:** This is common in babies, especially those that are born after their due date. If this occurs, apply some baby oil/emollient to the skin.

Other conditions that are common to newborns are:

- **Birthmarks**: Quite commonly there are small red marks on the baby's skin, particularly on the forehead, upper eyelids and back of the neck (**stork marks**). They are due to enlargement of the tiny blood vessels near the surface of the skin. They tend to disappear within the first year of life. Another common birthmark is the **strawberry mark**. Though a birthmark, it may not be apparent at birth and only appear at one month in life. It tends to grow in size initially till about six months and then slowly fades. Ask your doctor for advice should your baby have one that is growing rapidly or tends to bleed.

- **Mongolian blue spots** are the blue-grey patches that can be found all over the body, but are especially common on the buttocks, back and limbs. 90% of Asian babies have Mongolian blue spots but few adults still do, which show us that these discolorations usually disappear with time.

Eye Discharge

Ensure that your baby is able to open both eyes, and that it is not so sticky that they are unable to open their eyes. Clean the eyes using a cotton ball soaked in cooled boiled water and wipe each eye outward away from the nose. Gentle massage around the eyes can help clear the ducts. If the eye discharge persists, the eyeball looks red or the eyelid swells then consult your doctor to rule out any infection.

Umbilical Cord Care

Immediately after birth, the umbilical cord is cut and the cord is clamped. The cord tends to dry up and drop off within ten days of life. Clean the cord using cooled boiled water and keep it dry. Fold the nappy below the cord stump, keeping the cord stump above the nappy so that the cord does not get wet when baby passes urine.

Umbilical Hernia

Some babies develop a bulge in the region of the umbilicus. This is a common condition that nearly always resolves on its own, usually within the year.

Jaundice

This is a common newborn condition. There are many causes. **Usually it develops on the third day of life,** and is known as **physiological jaundice**. It is due to the baby's blood having a high content of primitive red cells which are broken down after birth.

One of the breakdown products is **bilirubin**, which causes the yellow discoloration of skin and whites of the eye. Most infants have mild jaundice and this is harmless. **However in some infants, the bilirubin level can be very high and this may cause brain damage if not treated**. If your baby appears to have jaundice, get him assessed by your doctor. Your doctor may do a blood test to determine your baby's bilirubin level.

Depending on the result, your baby may require treatment with **phototherapy**, which uses specific ultra-violet light that help break down the harmful products of jaundice, which is then excreted in the urine and feces.

In some occasions, the level of jaundice can rise so high that phototherapy may not be effective. A special procedure known as **exchange transfusion** might then be necessary.

Jaundice can sometimes last for about two weeks, especially if your child is breastfed. (Breast milk is still the ideal food for your baby though.)

If your child is still jaundiced more than two weeks after birth, then consult your doctor who will review your baby to see if any further tests are necessary, or to reassure you.

Which babies require more attention for jaundice?

Some babies are at a greater risk for high levels of jaundice. These **risk factors** include:

- Prematurity (less than 37 weeks)
- Jaundice that appears in the first 24 hours of life
- Breastfeeding that is not going well
- Bruising or bleeding under the scalp, which are related to labor and delivery
- Family history of jaundice (a parent or sibling who previously had high bilirubin levels that required treatment with phototherapy)
- G6PD deficiency
- Blood group incompatibility

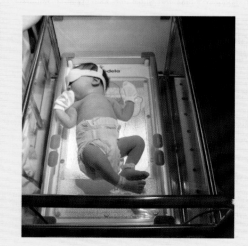

Figure 49.1 Baby undergoing phototherapy.

Crying Baby

Your baby cries as a form of communication. Once you get to know your baby, you will realize that their cry varies for different needs.

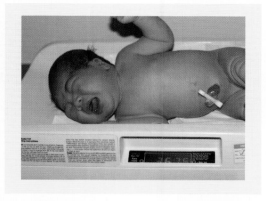

Sometimes they may cry for long periods, inconsolably. This may start from about two weeks of age and last till about four months of age, and is often referred to as **colic**. It often occurs in the evening but can occur at any time, and may last a few hours. It is a diagnosis of exclusion when no identifiable cause is found, and your baby appears very well in between these crying bouts. Consult your doctor to rule out any possibility that your baby is unwell. Once reassured, try and keep calm in the knowledge that it will all resolve in a few months and that there will be no permanent damage.

Infections

Your newborn baby's immune system is less developed than an older child, so sometimes a mild illness in an adult may result in a serious infection. However, for about the first six months of life, your baby has the benefit of protection from some illnesses as they have their mother's antibodies. But be sensible! Do not put your baby in a situation where you cannot adequately control the environment around you, for example, a crowded place, till your baby's immune status is at least "old enough" to fight off these germs. Remember to immunize your child, as this is the surest way of ensuring that they have some protection against some infectious diseases.

Stools

Baby's stools always seem to be a source of worry for parents. Your baby's first stools are usually sticky, tarry and dark green or almost black in color. This is called **meconium**. Within the next few days, your baby's stools will slowly change color and consistency. Stool color can vary from green, yellow to brown and these are all normal. The number of times that your baby passes stools will also vary. Generally, breastfed babies tend to pass softer and more frequent stools than formula fed babies. As babies get older, they pass stools less frequently. It is normal for some babies to pass stools many times a day in the first few weeks of life and for the pattern to change so that they only pass motion once every 2–3 days.

Review at 4 to 6 Weeks

At 4–6 weeks, your baby is usually reviewed again by their doctor. They will assess baby's growth, behavioral development and overall state of health.

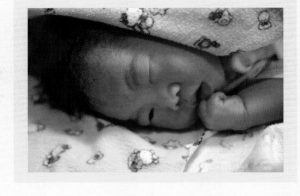

At 6 weeks, your baby will start to

- smile responsively
- stare at their parents' face and even start to follow when you move
- will startle to sound
- start to control their head a little bit more.

While you feed, carry and even change your baby's diapers, this is time spent bonding with your child. You gain confidence in handling your child and you and your baby get to know each other. Soon you will start to recognize what is normal for your child.

If there is any doubt, always consult your doctor.

Enjoy this wondrous time that you have with your child.

Contact your doctor when your baby:

- Cries more than usual
- Screams as if in pain
- Is unusually quiet or drowsy
- Has diarrhoea or vomiting
- Has sunken or a bulging soft spot on the top of the head
- Breathes much faster than usual
- Has difficulty breathing
- Has fever
- Has cold, pale or clammy skin

Your baby will usually pass his/her first urine within the first 24 hours of age and his first stool within the first 1–2 days of age.

Chapter 50

Vaccination for Your Baby

> *A baby has a special way of adding joy in every single day.*
>
> **Anonymous**

Immunization is an important way to protect your child from certain life threatening diseases. All the diseases that your child is protected against are serious diseases and by immunizing your child, you are also ensuring better protection for the population.

How does Immunity Work?

We get sick when our bodies are invaded by germs. For example the measles virus enters the body and gives us measles. Our immune system is meant to protect us from these germs.

These germs enter our body and start to reproduce. Our immune system responds to these "invaders" by making proteins called **antibodies**. These antibodies help to destroy the germs that are making us sick. But as these germs have already been in our body, we would already feel sick by the time our immune system has produced enough antibodies to destroy them. However by eliminating the attacking germs, antibodies then help us get well. Antibodies also have another job. They remain in our bloodstream, guarding us against future infections. So if the same germs ever try to infect us again even after many years, these antibodies will come to our defense. Only now they can destroy the germs before they have a chance to make us sick. This process is called **immunity**. This is a very effective system to prevent future disease.

How Do Vaccines Help?

The idea behind vaccination is to give us immunity to a disease ***before it has a chance to make us sick***.

Vaccines are made from the same virus or bacterium (or parts of them) that cause disease. But in vaccines, they are altered so that they cannot cause illness. These vaccines containing the weakened or killed germs are introduced into our body, usually by injection. Our immune system reacts to the vaccine in the same way as the disease, by making antibodies. Then they stay in our body, giving us immunity and hence afford protection against those diseases.

This "immunologic memory" lasts longer for some vaccines than for others and sometimes re-vaccination is required to maintain protection. Immunizations therefore help the child's immune system do its work. The child develops protection against future infections, the same as if he or she had been exposed to the natural disease. The good news is, with vaccines your child does not have to get sick first to get that protection.

What are Some of the Diseases that are Preventable?

- **Tuberculosis (TB)** is caused by a bacteria that infects lungs, bones, brain, kidneys and intestines. We give the **BCG** at birth to protect against this disease.
- **Hepatitis B** is a virus that can lead to serious complications in adulthood, like chronic liver failure and even liver cancer.
- **Diphtheria** is a bacterial disease that starts in the throat and can cause obstruction to breathing and can also spread to the heart and nervous system.
- **Tetanus** is a bacterial disease that can get into the body from cuts in the skin. It produces a toxin in the body that begins with clamping together of the jaw, hence the old name "lockjaw". It can also cause severe muscle spasms of any muscles including that of respiration and swallowing, leading to death in about 10 % of cases.
- **Pertussis** (**Whooping cough**) is a bacterial infection that can cause coughing spasms that can result in vomiting, seizures, lung damage.and even death in some cases.
- **Poliomyelitis** was the dreaded childhood disease of the 20th century. Polio is a viral infection that can be transmitted easily through consuming contaminated water or food. It typically affects young children with majority occurring under three years of age. Most have mild symptoms like fever, sore throat, but if the virus enters the brain and spinal cord, disease may result in paralysis and death.
- *Hemophilus influenzae* **type B** is a bacteria that can cause serious, often life threatening infections like bacterial meningitis, pneumonia or epiglottis which affects the windpipe, and can lead to brain damage or death.

- **Measles** is a virus that can cause chest infections, severe ear infections that can result in deafness, seizures and even permanent brain damage.
- **Mumps** is caused by a virus, which causes painful swellings of the salivary gland and fever. Its complications include meningitis, encephalitis, painful swelling of the testicles, deafness, and even death.
- **Rubella** is caused by a virus that is usually mild in adults but if it occurs in early pregnancy, can lead to miscarriage and congenital rubella syndrome.
- **Chicken pox (*Varicella zoster*)** is caused by a virus, which is spread by air-droplets and direct contact with fluid from blisters. It is contagious from 1–2 days before rash appears till 5–7 days later when it is totally dry. It is usually a mild irritating illness in the acute phase, but it can lead to serious complications like scarring, pneumonia, encephalitis and shingles.
- ***Streptococcus pneumoniae*** is a bacteria that is spread through respiratory droplets. It can cause pneumonia, bacteraemia and meningitis (especially in the < 5 year olds).
- **Rotavirus** causes severe gastroenteritis (vomiting and diarrhea) in infants and young children worldwide.

In Singapore, the National Childhood Immunization Programme is based on recommendations from Singapore's National Vaccine advisory committee and the World Health Organization. It is made up of the Childhood Vaccination Program, which is conducted by the Family Health Service, hospitals and clinics; and the School Vaccination Program which is conducted by the School Health Service.

Childhood Vaccination Program

Time of vaccination	Vaccine
Birth	Hep B (Hepatitis B) 1st dose
	BCG (Bacillus Calmette-Guerin)
1 month	Hep B 2nd dose
3 months	DTP-Polio (Diphtheria, Tetanus, Pertussis-Polio) 1st dose
4 months	DTP-Polio 2nd dose
5 months	DTP-Polio 3rd dose
6 months	Hep B 3rd dose
12–24 months	MMR (Measles, Mumps, Rubella) 1st dose
18 months	DTP-Polio 1st booster

School Health Program

Time of vaccination	Vaccine
6–7 yrs	– oral polio – 2nd booster – MMR – booster
10–11 yrs	– DT – 2nd booster – oral polio – 3rd booster

Currently, some of these vaccines have been combined into a single vaccine so your baby can get the benefit of all these vaccines, and yet not require multiple injections. In other words, your child still gains the same protection from the vaccines, but there are fewer injections involved to achieve the same protection.

There are also additional vaccines that are available, these include vaccines against chicken-pox, Haemophilus Influenzae B (Hib) bacterial infection, Streptococcus Pneumoniae and Rotavirus.

Common Types of Combination Vaccines Available in Singapore

Combination vaccine	Example
Diphtheria, Tetanus, Pertussis	Infanrix (GSK)
Diphtheria, Tetanus, acellular Pertussis	Boostrix (GSK) aka 3-in-1
Diphtheria, Tetanus, acellular Pertussis, Polio, H. influenzae	Infanrix-IPV + HiB (GSK) aka 5-in-1
Diphtheria, Tetanus, acellular Pertussis, Polio, H. influenzae, Hepatitis B	Infanrix Hexa (GSK) aka 6-in-1

Well Baby Vaccination Schedule Available in KKH

Time of vaccination	Vaccine
At birth	BCG, Hepatitis B
2 months	Diphtheria, Tetanus, acellular Pertussis, Polio, H. Influenzae, Hepatitis B (Hexa)
4 months	Diphtheria, Tetanus, acellular Pertussis, Polio, H. Influenzae (5-in-1)
6 months	Diphtheria, Tetanus, acellular Pertussis, Polio, H. Influenzae, Hepatitis B (Hexa)
15 months	Measles, Mumps, Rubella (MMR), Varicella (Chicken pox)
18 months	Diphtheria, Tetanus, acellular Pertussis, Polio, H. Influenzae (5-in-1)
Optional	Pneumococcus Vaccine, Rotavirus Vaccine

If you have any concerns/queries about immunizations, please discuss this with your doctor.

When to delay immunization

- When your baby is born prematurely and weighs less than 2 kg.
- When the child is unwell, for example a high fever, then delay the immunization till the child is better.
- If the child is being assessed for a neurological problem, is being treated for cancer or has any disease that weakens the immune system, discuss this with your child's doctor.
- Speak with your doctor if your child has had a serious reaction to any previous injection or has an allergy to eggs or anything else.

Side effects of vaccines

The needle does cause brief pain, so it is normal for your baby to cry a little. Often this is just for a few seconds after the injection. Soreness, a slight redness and even a small lump are common, but this usually resolves on its own. It is also normal for a child to be a little more irritable for a few hours or even a day or so after the injection and there may also be a slight fever ($<38°C$) that tends to last usually 1–2 days.

Your doctor may prescribe a small dose of paracetamol for pain or fever.

Chapter 51

Resuming Sexual Relations and Contraception

> *You may delay, but time will not.*
>
> **Benjamin Franklin**

Love Life After Giving Birth

Making sacrifices is part of parenthood. But that does not mean that you have to give up your love life.

Indeed, trying to meet the new demands of caring for your newborn as well as spending time to become an intimate couple can be difficult. It is important that you focus on your own and your partner's needs as well.

Good and strong relationships are based on trust and understanding. Being open and honest which each other is crucial. If you are too caught up with your new duties as a mother and feel the intense pressure, do confide with your partner. If you are worried that sexual intercourse will hurt, talk to your partner about what feels good and what hurts. Keep an open communication and he will definitely understand.

Resume Your Love Life

Most women are able to resume sex after six weeks as it usually takes four to six weeks for your body to recover from delivery. However, there is no fixed time frame when you will actually start feeling the mood again. It varies from one woman to another.

If you find that you are not in the mood for sexual intercourse yet, try to explore other ways of intimacy, for example, snuggling, kissing or caressing.

Tips to Get into the Right Mood

- Take time to do things that make you feel good about your body. It could be a long soak in the tub, getting your hair done or going for a leisure walk outdoors. Feeling relaxed and good about yourself make a huge difference.

- Find time to be alone with your partner and enjoy the opportunity. (Getting a trusted friend or family member to baby-sit so that you do not have to spend the entire time worrying can really help things progress!)
- If you are nervous about making love, try easing into it slowly. Date each other for romantic outings. Start with just kissing, then gradually progress to touching and so on until you are ready for sex.

Sex Can Be Good for You

It is easy for new parents to adopt the attitude that sex is a luxury for those with lots of free time and energy on their hands — like all your childless friends. But the fact is, having sex can be really good for you!

- **Sex helps to de-stress**
  Sex is one of the most effective forms of stress relief — plus it is natural.
- **Sex is a great exercise**
  Making love three times a week burns around 7,500 calories in a year — that is equivalent to jogging for 75 miles.
- **Production of natural hormones**
  Regular lovemaking can increase a woman's estrogen level, which is important to keep her bones strong and improve the suppleness of her vaginal tissues.
- **Increased oxygenation**
  All that heavy breathing increases the amount of oxygen in the cells, helping to keep organs and tissues functioning properly.
- **Pain relief**
  Sex reduces arthritic pain, whiplash pain and headaches. What is more, the hormones that are released during sexual arousal and orgasm can actually elevate your pain threshold.
- **Bonding**
  Affectionate touching increases your level of oxytocin — also known as the "bonding" hormone.

TEN Tips to Get You Back into Action

- **Environment**
  A romantic atmosphere can set the right mood for intimacy.

- **Relax**
  Find ways to relax before trying to make love (for example, taking a shower together or exchanging massages).
- **Lubricate**
  Lowered hormone levels after pregnancy can make the vagina tissue dry and uncomfortable. To avoid painful intercourse, use lubricating gel until your natural secretions return.
- **Warm up**
  Do not rush into sex. The more foreplay you can fit in, the better.
- **Minimize distractions**
  Turn off both your cell phones. This is your private time, so enjoy it.
- **Experiment**
  Some positions give the woman more control over penetration and put less pressure on an episiotomy site or cesarean scar (eg. side-to-side or woman-on-top positions).
- **Be realistic**
  Some women may not experience orgasms at all for several weeks after childbirth or orgasms may be a little delayed in coming.
- **Communicate**
  Let your partner know what feels good and what does not.
- **Make time to make love**
  While life has become more hectic with a newborn in the house, do not let lovemaking disappear from your lives. Take time to be intimate with your partner.
- **Do not worry**
  You may feel like you will never be passionate about sex again. This is not true as it is only a temporary state of mind.

Planning for the Next Pregnancy

While some couples believe in letting nature take its course, others may prefer to plan the timing of their subsequent pregnancies. Whatever your inclination may be, remember that what works for someone else may not necessarily be the best choice for you. Your circumstances are unique and should be taken into consideration.

Some practical aspects that you should consider carefully before getting pregnant again include your financial status, your emotional and physical well-being and your partner's preference. There is no absolute right or wrong in your decision. There are both pros and cons in spacing your children closer together or farther apart.

Having children with ages farther apart

Advantages

- By the time your next child is due, the earlier one is old enough to do certain things on his or her own, relieving you of much stress.
- You can focus your time on one child before having another.
- You can have a recovery time before going through another pregnancy. Your body needs to replenish its store of nutrients (for example, calcium and iron stores).

Disadvantages

- It may be difficult to attend to the different needs of a younger and an older child at the same time.
- Your children may not share similar interests because of their age difference and may have difficulty playing together.
- The older child may feel that he or she has lost your attention and love to the younger one.

Having children with ages close together

Advantages

- You can focus on similar needs of your children at the same time.
- You spend less number of years in bringing up your children.
- Children who are closer in age share similar interests and are often great playmates.

Disadvantages

- You need to put in more energy in providing special care to more than one child during their early and crucial years.

Contraception — What are Your Options?

Your fertility can return within weeks after giving birth. Although your body may have barely recovered from childbirth, you may get pregnant when you have sex unless you are fully breastfeeding. If you are fully breastfeeding and your menses have not resumed, you are protected from pregnancy (1–2% risk failure rate though). This is known as lactational amenorhoea method (LAM).

It is therefore important that you use contraception as soon as you start having sex again if you do not want an unplanned pregnancy.

There are many reliable methods of contraception. Some are suitable for breast feeding (Table 51.1) while others are not (Table 51.2). Some women may not be suitable for certain types of contraception. For example, those women with a history of breast cancer should not take the pill while women with a history of pelvic infection are not suitable for intra-uterine copper device.

Most methods of contraception are reversible and most women will get pregnant within six months of stopping contraception. The irreversible or permanent method like sterilization or ligation must be considered carefully (Table 51.3). We do not recommend any woman under the age of 35 to undergo the permanent methods as they may regret in future and may not be able to bear another kid again unless they go for reversal surgery or assisted reproductive techniques (test-tube baby).

Please discuss with your doctor regarding the contraceptive method that is most suitable for you.

Table 51.1 Contraception suitable for breastfeeding.

Methods	Reliability (Success rate)	Contraceptive duration	Reversibility	How to use
Levonorgestrel releasing intrauterine system (IUS)	Very high (99.8%)	5 years	Yes	One time insertion six weeks after delivery. Short and light periods.
Copper intrauterine device (IUD)	High (99.5%)	3 or 5 years (depends on type)	Yes	One time insertion six weeks after delivery
Mini pill	High/ Moderate (96–99%)	Daily	Yes	Take daily
Male condom / Female diaphragm	High/ Moderate (85–96%)	Per usage	Yes	Must use before penetration. Effectiveness depends on correct technique of usage.
Hormonal injectable	High/ Moderate (98–99%)	Monthly or 3-monthly injectables	Yes	May cause irregular periods

Table 51.2 Contraception if you are not breastfeeding.

Methods	Reliability (Success rate)	Contraceptive duration	Reversibility	How to use
Oral combined pills	High/ very high (97–99.8%)	As used	Yes	Daily oral pills for three weeks and one week of "pill holiday". (Modern pills do not have the water-retention related weight gain and acne).

Table 51.3 Irreversible or permanent methods of contraception.

Methods	Reliability (Success rate)	Contraceptive duration	Reversibility	How to use
Female sterilization (See *Figure 51.1*)	High (99.5%)	Permanent	No (If fertility is still desired, the woman has to undergo surgical reversal of the ligation or test-tube baby (in vitro fertilization).)	Involves permanent blockage of fallopian tubes with clips or cutting segments of tubes under general anesthesia. Can be done immediately after delivery via a mini-incision (post-partum sterilization or PPS). Or at least six weeks after delivery via key-hole surgery (laparoscopy). This method has a lower failure rate than PPS as the tubes are swollen immediately after delivery and the clips have an increased risk of slippage.
Male sterilisation (vasectomy)	Most effective (99.95%)	Permanent	No	Involves cutting or tying of vas deferens of male partner.

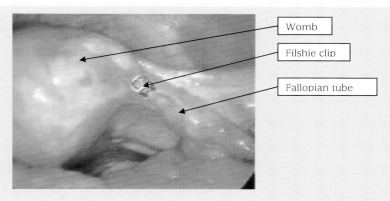

Womb

Filshie clip

Fallopian tube

Figure 51.1 Permanent female sterilization with Filshie clip on the fallopian tube.

FREQUENTLY ASKED QUESTIONS

1. **What are the contraceptive options for women during the post-partum phase?**

   Mothers, who are fully breastfeeding and have no menses yet, are protected from pregnancy in the first six months. This is known as lactational amenorrhoea method (LAM). Others use barrier methods like condoms. These women who are breastfeeding can also decide on hormonal methods like mini pills and injectables. Another option is the intra-uterine device, which is inserted into the womb six weeks after delivery. Oral contraceptive pills can be used if the woman chooses **not to breastfeed**.

   Some couples choose **permanent sterilization** such as female fallopian tubal ligation/cutting or male sterilization/vasectomy (tying of vas deferens).

2. **What is the efficacy and side effect profile of each option?**

   Lactational Amenorrhoea Method has a failure rate of 1–2%. There is no side effect as this is a natural contraception.

   Hormonal methods are highly effective with a failure rate of less than 1%. The disadvantage of the **mini pill** is that it has to be taken daily and at around the same time of the day. This requires strong motivation and compliance. **Injectables** are convenient and given every three months. However, it causes irregular menstrual spotting which can be irritating. Some women develop depression and weight gain as well. **Oral contraceptive pills (OCP)** can be used for **non-breastfeeding mothers** and may interfere with breast milk production. It can worsen migraine in some women and rarely causes deep vein thrombosis (blood clots) in the legs.

Intrauterine device is also effective with failure of less than 1%. However, it may cause pelvic pain and infection in some women and the insertion can result in womb perforation occasionally.

Condoms are dependent on the correct technique of usage and has failure rate of 4–15%. It disrupts the sexual experience as condoms have to be worn before penetration and removed immediately after ejaculation. However, it is the only protection against sexually transmitted diseases.

Natural methods like rhythm and withdrawal methods are least effective with failure rates of 30%. There is no side effect though.

Permanent sterilization is irreversible. Failure of tubal ligation is 1 in 200 women while failure of vasectomy is 1 in 2000. Besides, tubal ligation carries surgical risks and risk of ectopic pregnancy (outside the womb) if the contraception fails.

3. **Are there any special precautions that women should take into account while choosing a contraceptive method during the postpartum stage?**

When choosing a birth control method, it is always necessary to weigh the advantages and disadvantages. Consideration must be given to the effectiveness and the potential side effects as well as your individual circumstances, health, age and personal/partner's preferences.

The method you choose also depends on when you plan for the next baby or if you have completed your family (i.e. may choose permanent methods). Besides, your decision for breastfeeding also affects your contraceptive choice.

Your doctor is an important partner in helping you choose the suitable form of contraception, but he/she cannot make the decision for you. Discuss with him/her!

4. **Which is the most popular contraceptive method in Singapore?**

In a population survey conducted by the Obstetrical and Gynecological Society of Singapore in 2006, only 47% of women in the reproductive age group used any form of contraception. Of those who used contraception, 47% used condoms and 21% used withdrawal or rhythm method. Only 13% tried the pills or injectables. 12% chose permanent sterilization while the remaining 7% used intra-uterine contraceptive device (IUCD).

5. Are there any new contraceptives available, or any new products or devices which will be available in the near future?

The ideal contraceptive, which is 100% effective with no side effects and suitable for all age groups, has yet to be discovered. We will continue to work on it!

6. I had unprotected sex last night and am worried about getting pregnant. What should I do?

There 2 types of emergency contraception such as "morning-after pill" and use of copper intrauterine contraceptive device (IUCD).

The morning-after pill consists of two **large** doses of hormonal pills. The **first dose** must be taken **within 72 hours of unprotected or inadequately protected intercourse**, followed by a **second dose 12 hours later**. It is meant only as a **back-up method** of birth control to be used on an **emergency basis only**. On the other hand, **copper IUCD** can also be inserted for suitable patients **up to 5 days of unprotected intercourse**.

7. Are there risks if I use emergency contraception on a regular basis?

The side-effects of high-dose hormonal pills are nausea and vomiting, irregular menses in the next period and breast tenderness. If the morning-after pill fails, there is an increased risk of tubal ectopic pregnancy. Also, the "morning-after pill" has a failure **rate of 10–20%** and thus will not be advised as a regular contraceptive method.

Chapter 52

Common Urinary Problems and Womb Prolapse

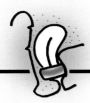

" Hope is the expectation that something outside of ourselves, something or someone external, is going to come to our rescue and we will live happily ever after. "

Dr Robert Anthony

Introduction

The female bladder stores and passes urine at the appropriate time and place. When there are problems with bladder function, the patient will need to visit the toilet often, unable to pass urine or even leak urine. On the other hand, prolapse of the pelvic organs such as the urinary bladder (urine "bag"), womb, and rectum (back-passage) is very common and occurs in more than 10% of women.

Urinary Frequency and Urgency

Urinary frequency is the need to pass urine for more than seven times during the day or less than every 2 hourly.

Urgency is a strong and sudden desire to void which, if not relieved immediately, may lead to urge incontinence.

Urge Incontinence is an involuntary leakage of urine, usually preceded by urgency.

What are the common causes of frequency and urgency?

Classification	Causes
Psychosocial	Excessive drinking Habit Anxiety
Urological	Urinary tract infection Detrusor (bladder muscle) overactivity Bladder tumor Bladder stones
Gynecological	Pregnancy Bladder prolapse Pelvic mass, e.g. fibroids
Medical	Diuretic therapy Diseases of the brain/spinal cord Diabetes

What to do if you have urinary frequency and urgency?

You should visit you family doctor. The doctor will then ask you a few questions on your medical history and urinary habits. After a physical examination, he/she may perform a few simple tests such as collecting your urine specimen for analysis to **exclude urinary tract infection**. Depending on the cause of your condition, the doctor may start you on medication or refer you to a specialist for further management.

Urinary Incontinence

Urinary incontinence refers to an **involuntary loss of urine**. Types of incontinence includes:

- **Stress urinary incontinence** — involuntary loss of urine associated with coughing, sneezing, carrying heavy things and even running or jumping.
- **Urge incontinence** — involuntary loss of urine preceded by a sudden strong desire to pass urine and voiding before the ability to reach the toilet.
- **Overflow incontinence** — involuntary loss of urine due to an inability to empty the bladder well.

What should you do if you have urinary incontinence?

Mild urinary incontinence may not be troublesome but moderate to severe urinary incontinence can affect the quality of life of the woman drastically. It can also cause social and hygiene problems.

Table 52.1 Management of incontinence.

Types of incontinence	Management	Comments
Stress urinary incontinence	Pelvic floor exercises	This is helpful in mild stress incontinence with success rate of 50%–60%.
	Continence surgery	There are many types of continence procedures but the gold standard is the **suburethral sling procedure** (Figure 52.1). It involves a minimally invasive procedure, which can be performed as a day surgery procedure. Its success rate is about 90%.
Urge incontinence	Oral medication	Medication will relieve the symptoms in 80%–90%.
Overflow incontinence	May require clean intermittent draining of urine or placement of continuous urine catheter (tube).	May be prone to urinary infection.

These women should seek help from their doctor. Management depends on the type of incontinence and the severity of the condition.

Management of urinary incontinence

Regular pelvic floor exercises can be performed to improve the incontinence for **mild cases**. In **severe cases** of stress urinary incontinence, **surgical correction** by your gynecologist should be considered (Table 52.1).

Urinary Tract Infection (UTI)

UTI is due to the **presence of bacteria in the urine**. UTI can be divided into either **upper tract infection (kidney)** or **lower tract infection (bladder)**.

   Pyelonephritis is the acute bacterial infection of the kidneys. Patients have severe back pain and high fever. There may be presence of frequency and urgency of urine as well. **Cystitis** is the infection of

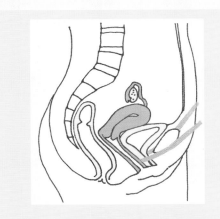

Figure 52.1 Suburethral sling procedure.

the urinary bladder and patients complain of frequency, urgency and dysuria (pain on passing urine).

What should you do if you have a urinary tract infection (UTI)?

General measures for simple cystitis include taking more fluids of more than two liters a day to encourage more urine formation to flush out the bacteria.

You would need to consult a doctor if the symptoms persist or if you have a fever. **Oral antibiotics** prescribed by the doctor would eradicate 90% of infection in a normal person. The doctor may order some investigations relevant to your condition if necessary.

Patients having **severe UTI** associated with fever and kidney infection **may require intravenous antibiotics and hospitalization**.

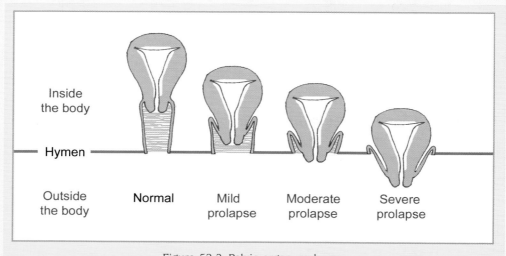

Figure 52.2 Pelvic organ prolapse.

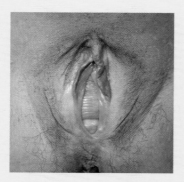

Figure 52.3 Mild womb prolapse.

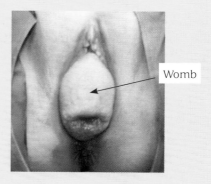

Figure 52.4 Severe womb prolapse.

Uterovaginal Prolapse

What is uterovaginal prolapse (UVP)?

This is the protrusion of the pelvic organs (bladder, uterus and rectum) down into or out of the vagina. Patients usually complain of feeling something heavy at the vagina or sensation of a lump protruding out of the introitus. There are different degrees of severity as shown in the diagram below (Figures 52.2, 52.3 and 52.4).

What are the causes of uterovaginal prolapse (UVP)?

- Vaginal delivery of baby
- Pregnancy
- Heavy lifting
- Chronic constipation
- Menopause

How can I prevent uterovaginal prolapse (UVP)?

The risks of UVP may be **reduced** by

- Pelvic floor exercises **during** pregnancy and **after** vaginal delivery (see Chapter 18)
- Avoiding carrying heavy objects
- Treating chronic constipation
- Maintaining body weight in the healthy range

Management of uterovaginal prolapse (UVP)

The patient complains of a lump at the introitus. She would not be able to differentiate whether the protruding organ is the bladder (cystocele), womb or rectum (rectocele). The doctor needs to perform a pelvic examination to ascertain the site and degree of the prolapse.

Conservative measures include using **a ring pessary and local hormone therapy**. However, the use of the ring pessary may be associated with vaginal infection or ulceration of the vagina leading to vaginal discharge or bleeding.

Surgery is presently **the treatment of choice for pelvic organ prolapse** unless patient is not fit for surgery.

Conservation of the uterus is possible if the patient chooses to keep her womb.

Chapter 53

Traditional Chinese Medicine (TCM) and Confinement

> *The greatest wealth is health.*
>
> **Virgil**

The postnatal period or confinement is a critical time for new mothers to adapt and recuperate their health. As this may be a totally new experience for some mothers, much energy is channeled into feeding and taking care of the newborn. Thus, many new mothers may find little time to care for themselves and hence conditions such as insomnia, fatigue or depression may be easily triggered.

In Traditional Chinese Medicine (TCM), the confinement period is crucial for the mother's body system, which had just undergone the physical demands of pregnancy and labor, to recuperate.

Some Common Postnatal Conditions in TCM

Lochiorrhea（恶露不绝）

Lochia refers to vaginal discharge after delivery of baby. This usually consists of blood, debris, leukocytes (white blood cells) and serous (watery) fluids from the womb in the first two weeks after childbirth. Lochiorrhea is excessive amount of lochia especially after more than three weeks of childbirth. Lochiorrhea must be treated as soon as possible to prevent excessive loss of blood that may lead to anemia.

In TCM, it is believed that lochiorrhea may be due to the loss of huge amounts of Qi and Blood during labor. In Qi deficiency (气虚), TCM aims to replenish and nourish Qi and restore the blood loss. Lochiorrhoea could also be due to the internal heat build-up in the body (内热扰胞宫). Thus, treatment is to nourish the "yin" to clear away the accumulated internal heat.

Postpartum hypogalactia（乳汁不行/缺乳）

This is defined as abnormally low milk secretion that is insufficient to breast-feed the newborn. As Qi is embedded in the Blood, much of this Qi is depleted through Blood lost during delivery. This condition can be worsened with the malfunctioning of the Spleen, which takes care of the work of generating sufficient Qi and Blood. It is important to distinguish hypogalactia from diminished milk secretion due to blocked ducts of the nipples.

In TCM, the causes of postpartum hypogalactia are listed below.

1. <u>Qi and Blood deficiency</u>（气血虚弱）

Main symptoms:
- a. Lack of milk secretions after childbirth
- b. Poor appetite
- c. Dull complexion
- d. Pale tongue with little or no tongue coat
- e. Weak but deep intense pulse

Suggested TCM therapeutic methodology:
- – Nourishing Qi and Blood to improve the ability to lactate.

2. <u>Stagnation of Liver Qi</u>（肝郁气滞）

Main symptoms:
- a. Lack of milk secretions after childbirth
- b. Swollen, hardness or pain sensation felt in the breasts
- c. Distended sensation felt in the chest region
- d. Poor appetite
- e. May develop mild fever
- f. Taut, deep intense but rapid pulse

Suggested TCM therapeutic methodology:
- – Improve collateral circulation to promote milk secretions.
- – Relieve stagnation to alleviate the pain.

Granny's Recipe for Confinement

There are some recipes from our grandmothers, which have been used over decades to ensure a smooth and pleasant confinement period for new mothers.

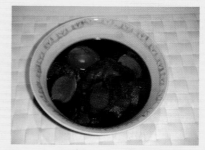

Figure 53.1 Pig trotters in black vinegar.

Pig Trotters in Black Vinegar Recipe

Ingredients:

1 pair of pig trotters	600 g of brown sugar
1 kg of matured ginger	4 hard-boiled eggs
6 tablespoons of sesame seed oil	9 cups of water
4 cups of black vinegar	

Instructions:

1. Clean the pig trotters and chop into big cubes.
2. Heat the sesame oil, add in ginger and fry till golden brown.
3. Place the fried ginger in a big clay pot and stir in vinegar, sugar and water.
4. Bring to boil and leave to simmer for about half an hour.
5. Add the pig's trotters and continue to simmer until the meat is tender.
6. Add the egg about 30 minutes before serving.
7. Best served warm.

Chinese Herbal Bath

Ingredients:

Artemesia argyi（艾叶）	30 g
Eucommia ulmoides（杜仲）	20 g
Ledebouriella divaricata（防风）	20 g
Perilla frutescens（紫苏叶）	20 g

Function: Improves blood circulation in new mothers.

Instructions:

1. Put the first three herbs in a muslin bag and seal.
2. Then put the herbs in a water kettle and bring to boil.
3. After boiling, discard the herbs and pour the water into the bath tub. Add same amount of hot water to fill the tub.
4. If bathtub is not available, the boiled decoction can be used to soak the feet or simply by rinsing or wiping the body with the herbal solution.
5. Note: This prescription is **not** suitable for mothers with fever after labor.

FREQUENTLY ASKED QUESTIONS

1. **Can I consume *Essence of Chicken* during confinement?**
   Essence of Chicken is made from chicken and contains no stimulants. It may improve absorption of iron and thus, restore your blood hemoglobin quicker. Also, it may help to reduce physical and mental fatigue.

2. **Can I consume *Lingzhi (Ganoderma Lucidum)* during confinement?**
   Lingzhi helps in the recovery after childbirth and is useful for insomnia or fatigue in new mothers. Due to the different species and product forms (e.g. capsules, tablets, powdered herbs) of Lingzhi, it is strongly recommended to consult a licensed TCM physician before consumption if you are breastfeeding.

Chapter 54

Myths about Confinement

> *The greatest achievement was at first and for a time a dream. The oak sleeps in the acorn; the bird waits in the egg; and in the highest vision of the soul a waking angel stirs. Dreams are the seedlings of realities.*
>
> **James Allen**

Confinement is a period for your body to recuperate and recover from childbirth. The idea of confinement is familiar to Asians but foreign to Westerners. In the past when infant and maternal mortality rates were high, it was a practice to keep both baby and mother indoors during the period of confinement. This was meant to protect mother and baby from ill health.

By now, you may have been exposed to some of the practices or ideas from your parents. You may or may not agree with them but many of these have originated from our Asian culture and hence, possess no scientific basis at all. They range from the prohibition of doing certain daily tasks to the restriction of certain food intake — with the strong belief that these can provide adequate rest and replenishment during this period.

	Chinese practices	Malay practices	Indian practices
Confinement Period	30 days	44 days	40 days
Dietary Requirements	• To purge out the "wind" in the body after delivery, promote "blood circulation", strengthen the joints and promote milk supply • To avoid "cooling" foods		
	Traditionally, they use a lot of ginger, wines and sesame oils in their diet. Common dishes include pigs trotters cooked with ginger and vinegar, fish soup, chicken cooked in sesame oil and a traditional tonic brewed from 10 herbs. Fish soup boiled with papaya is believed to be beneficial for milk production. It is also recommended that plain water consumption be avoided during this period to reduce the risk of water retention. Instead, specially prepared drinks from a mixture of herbs and preserved dates are recommended.	During confinement a woman follows a special diet in which heating foods are encouraged and cooling foods avoided to restore the balance upset by the birth. Some Malay mothers who have just delivered often take a special drink called "jamu". It is believed that the pores on the body are opened during labor and "jamu" has properties that can keep the body warm.	The Indians take garlic milk to prevent "wind". Like the Chinese and Malays, "cooling" foods are avoided, especially tomatoes, cucumbers, coconut milk and mutton. Only chicken and shark fish cooked with herbs are allowed while other seafood is not allowed. Chilli is not allowed. Plenty of garlic fried without oil is encouraged. Cooking is done with gingly oil. Oral intake of herbs or D.O.M. is encouraged to keep the body warm. There is restriction on fluids/fruits/vegetable intake as well as cold drinks and food.
Other Practices	The basis for such practices is to protect the new mother from future ill health, restore her strength and to protect the family from ritual pollution.		
	The Chinese believe in staying indoors throughout the confinement period to avoid outdoor pollution. Strenuous physical activities are discouraged to prevent further "muscle weakening".	Traditionally, childbirth is in the mother's home attended by a bidan (Malay midwife) and the umbilical stump dusted with a mixture of spices. Fortunately, this has been replaced by hospital births that reduce complications and infection rates.	Indian mothers are also discouraged from leaving their homes during their confinement period.

	Chinese practices	Malay practices	Indian practices
Other Practices	Some would hire a confinement nanny to help with the housework and caring for the baby. Other practices may include: • Not washing the body or hair during the month; especially avoiding contact with cold water. • Not going outside for the entire month (or at least avoid wind). • Not eating raw or "cooling" foods or foods cooked the previous day. • Eat chicken, especially chicken cooked in sesame oil; pork liver and kidney are also good; eat five or six meals daily and rinse the rice bowl with scalding water. • Avoid all wind, fans and air conditioning. • Avoid walking or moving about; the ideal is lying on the back in bed. • Do not go into another person's home. • Do not get sick. • Do not read or cry. • Do not have sex. • Do not eat with family members. • Do not burn incense or visit a temple or altar.	Both mother and child should be bathed immediately in heated water filled with herbs after birth. The mother will "keep warm" through various traditional methods. These may include sitting near to or lying above a heated source or warming the abdomen by applying a heated stone over it. During this confinement period, a female masseuse is engaged to help the mother regain her figure or at least to keep her extended tummy trim. The practice of tightly binding the tummy is called *berbengkong*, and is believed to help in maintaining the body shape. Sex is also strictly prohibited during the confinement period.	Bathing is discouraged and if done, it should be performed with special herbal preparations and turmeric powder. Bathing is only allowed between 11 am and 2 pm when the temperature is at its highest. Daily body massages with oil are also encouraged. • Not allowed to enter the prayer altar room. • Splashing of warm water on abdomen during bathing to expel clots from uterus. • Washing of hair is done on odd days i.e. day 3,5,7... during the first two weeks. Dry hair after washing with incense smoke. • Place incense smoke in between legs to dry episiotomy wound. • Binding of tummy with six feet cloth • Sex is strictly prohibited.

Let us now examine some of these myths in detail:

Myths	Medical perspective
"Now that my baby is born, I will lapse into depression."	It is true that most women experience a sad/depressed mood, beginning some days after the birth of the baby and continuing for varying lengths of time. These symptoms are termed the 'baby or postnatal blues' and are believed to be associated with hormonal changes following the birth of a child. Fortunately, it is of a relatively short-term duration (about two weeks) and most women recover from it. Depression is diagnosed only when these symptoms persist in a small proportion of women. It may be accompanied by suicidal or infanticide intent. Prompt psychiatric attention is imperative in such instances.
"I am not allowed to bath or touch water for fear of 'wind' entering the body." "I can only wash my hair with water in which ginger has been boiled in it."	There is no basis to this at all. In fact, bathing regularly ensures a good personal hygiene and comfort level. It reduces the incidence of skin and wound infections. On a personal note, it certainly ensures that people around you would find it more bearable.
"I must consume plenty of wines, sesame oils and traditional herbs to drive out the 'wind'".	Again, there is no medical reasoning behind this recommendation. In moderation, there is no harm in consuming these substances. However, when taken in excessive amounts, it may affect you and your baby. Furthermore, there are various substances present in the herbs that we are not fully aware of. Alcohol and other organic substances might go into your breast milk, and when breastfeeding, these might be transferred to your baby. These substances may affect the liver and worsen jaundice of the newborn if it is already present.
"I cannot drink plain water at all during confinement."	Adequate fluid consumption is advised especially if the mother is breastfeeding. The kidneys will produce more urine in the next few weeks after the baby is born to remove the excess fluid that has accumulated during the course of the pregnancy.
"I must not expose myself and the baby to any wind drafts or air-conditioner." "I must not leave my house for one month."	For personal comfort, there is definitely no harm in switching on the air-conditioner or fan, as long as it makes you and your baby comfortable. It may even help prevent heat rash from developing in our hot and humid climate.
"I must eat liver and meats only."	The confinement period is a time when physical changes that occurred in the last nine months will revert to the original state. It is also a period when nutritional demands on you are high, owing to the recent blood loss from the delivery and the demands of breastfeeding. The belief here is that the mother has been "cooled" by the delivery, and there is a need to eat "heating" foods such as meat. Many "confinement foods" have been devised to ensure that these nutritional demands and beliefs are met.

Myths	Medical perspective
"I must eat liver and meats only."	Whatever your beliefs are, it is important to take a well balanced diet than specific food types to replenish the body's stores. This is especially so during breastfeeding. If necessary, as in the case of vegetarians or vegans, iron or vitamin supplements may be taken to satisfy these nutritional demands.
"I have been told not to read or cry."	The traditional belief is that it causes eye problems later in life and this has no scientific logic.
"I cannot pray before an altar or enter a place of worship." "I cannot mingle with the rest of my family members or enter the kitchen."	Many believe that the post partum discharge (lochia) is unclean and therefore, this practice prevents any spiritual contamination. Again, there is no scientific basis to it.
"I heard that the Malay traditional practices are effective for regaining health."	There are six components to the traditional practices of postnatal care. These are: 1. *Tuku* — daily massage over the abdomen with a ball-like metal object 2. *Mengurut badan* — massaging by an experienced masseuse 3. *Barut* — tight wrap around the woman's waist 4. *Salai* — lying on a warmed wooden apparatus 5. *Air akar kayu* — tonic drinks made from medicinal plants 6. *Pantang makan dan minum* — to prohibit oneself from eating or drinking certain food items The main idea of the above is that specific massaging/heat/selective dieting helps promote blood circulation and recovery; while the *Barut* helps regain the woman's figure. Dieting to the Malays, like what the Chinese believe, ensures the avoidance of "cooling foods" and the intake of "heating foods". Although these practices have never been proven scientifically, it is possible that certain benefits can be derived from them. However, all these should be done in moderation to prevent burns and injuries from happening during these massages and therapies. **After a cesarean section, these have to be delayed for a month to prevent the disruption of a healing wound.** As mentioned previously, it is still essential to have a well-balanced diet to ensure adequate nutrition during this recovery period.
"Bathing should not be an issue."	This is prevalent in the Malay culture and is contrary to the Chinese practice. The water is warmed and herbs are added for a "heating effect". As mentioned before, this is good for personal hygiene and is encouraged.
"I cannot have sex for forty days."	This is against the religious teachings of certain cultures, e.g. the Malays. From a medical perspective, it allows for the lochia to be over and the episiotomy wound to be completely healed and this may reduce the incidence of infections.

Index

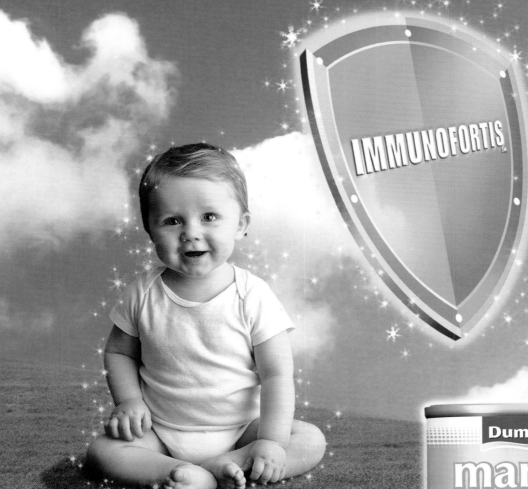
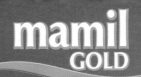
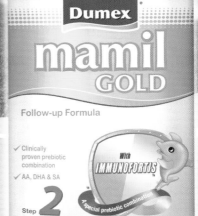

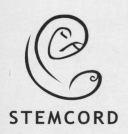

STEMCORD

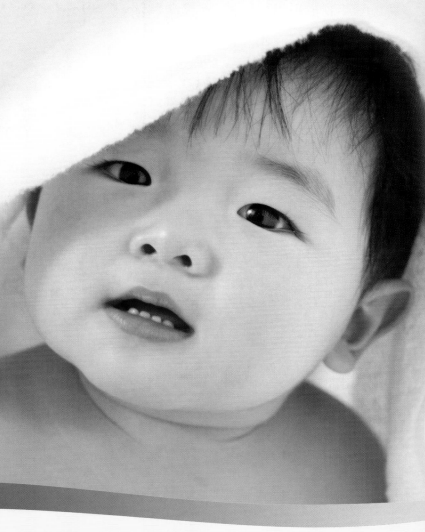

There's no *gift* more valuable than storing your **baby's cord blood.**

Preserving your newborn's umbilical cord blood is the best gift you can give to your child and family. That's because the blood in your newborn's umbilical cord is a rich source of stem cells which are precious as life-saving treatments for many disorders that could occur later in life.

You have only one opportunity to save your baby's cord blood, which is at birth. So act now for future peace of mind.

Find out more on Cord Blood Banking.

CALL: **6471 2002** for free home consultation and enquiries

SMS: **8222 4456** for free cord blood banking information kit
(Please indicate your address, expected date of delivery, hospital and doctor's name)

www.stemcord.com
StemCord Pte Ltd, Gleneagles Medical Centre 6 Napier Road #02-13 Singapore 258499

Want Strong
Healthy Bones?

Why Take Chances? Make Caltrate Part Of Your Life Today!

No Salt

No Sugar

No Lactose

No Preservatives

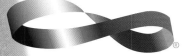

Caltrate®

Calcium Supplement

America's #1 Calcium Brand*

*IRI InfoScan data for 3 years from 2001 to Dec 2003

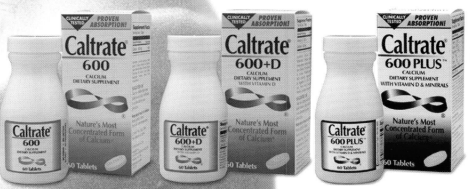

Caltrate, Food For Strong Bone